Saliva and Oral Diseases

Saliva and Oral Diseases

Editor

Pia Lopez-Jornet

MDPI • Basel • Beijing • Wuhan • Barcelona • Belgrade • Manchester • Tokyo • Cluj • Tianjin

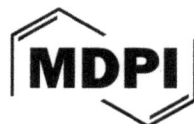

Editor
Pia Lopez-Jornet
Oral Medicine in the Department of Stomatology,
Faculty of Dentistry, University of Murcia
Spain

Editorial Office
MDPI
St. Alban-Anlage 66
4052 Basel, Switzerland

This is a reprint of articles from the Special Issue published online in the open access journal *Journal of Clinical Medicine* (ISSN 2077-0383) (available at: https://www.mdpi.com/journal/jcm/special_issues/saliva_oral).

For citation purposes, cite each article independently as indicated on the article page online and as indicated below:

LastName, A.A.; LastName, B.B.; LastName, C.C. Article Title. *Journal Name* **Year**, *Volume Number*, Page Range.

ISBN 978-3-0365-0776-7 (Hbk)
ISBN 978-3-0365-0777-4 (PDF)

© 2021 by the authors. Articles in this book are Open Access and distributed under the Creative Commons Attribution (CC BY) license, which allows users to download, copy and build upon published articles, as long as the author and publisher are properly credited, which ensures maximum dissemination and a wider impact of our publications.

The book as a whole is distributed by MDPI under the terms and conditions of the Creative Commons license CC BY-NC-ND.

Contents

About the Editor vii

Pia López Jornet
Special Issue "Saliva and Oral Diseases"
Reprinted from: *J. Clin. Med.* **2020**, *9*, 1955, doi:10.3390/jcm9061955 1

Piero Papi, Andrea Raco, Nicola Pranno, Bianca Di Murro, Pier Carmine Passarelli, Antonio D'Addona, Giorgio Pompa and Maurizio Barbieri
Salivary Levels of Titanium, Nickel, Vanadium, and Arsenic in Patients Treated with Dental Implants: A Case-Control Study
Reprinted from: *J. Clin. Med.* **2020**, *9*, 1264, doi:10.3390/jcm9051264 3

Pia Lopez-Jornet, Candela Castillo Felipe, Luis Pardo-Marin, Jose J. Ceron, Eduardo Pons-Fuster and Asta Tvarijonaviciute
Salivary Biomarkers and Their Correlation with Pain and Stress in Patients with Burning Mouth Syndrome
Reprinted from: *J. Clin. Med.* **2020**, *9*, 929, doi:10.3390/jcm9040929 13

Anna Skutnik-Radziszewska, Mateusz Maciejczyk, Iwona Flisiak, Julita Krahel, Urszula Kołodziej, Anna Kotowska-Rodziewicz, Anna Klimiuk and Anna Zalewska
Enhanced Inflammation and Nitrosative Stress in the Saliva and Plasma of Patients with Plaque Psoriasis
Reprinted from: *J. Clin. Med.* **2020**, *9*, 745, doi:10.3390/jcm9030745 23

Anna Zalewska, Agnieszka Kossakowska, Katarzyna Taranta-Janusz, Sara Zięba, Katarzyna Fejfer, Małgorzata Salamonowicz, Paula Kostecka-Sochoń, Anna Wasilewska and Mateusz Maciejczyk
Dysfunction of Salivary Glands, Disturbances in Salivary Antioxidants and Increased Oxidative Damage in Saliva of Overweight and Obese Adolescents
Reprinted from: *J. Clin. Med.* **2020**, *9*, 548, doi:10.3390/jcm9020548 41

Sanna Syrjäläinen, Ulvi Kahraman Gursoy, Mervi Gursoy, Pirkko Pussinen, Milla Pietiäinen, Antti Jula, Veikko Salomaa, Pekka Jousilahti and Eija Könönen
Salivary Cytokine Biomarker Concentrations in Relation to Obesity and Periodontitis
Reprinted from: *J. Clin. Med.* **2019**, *8*, 2152, doi:10.3390/jcm8122152 63

Fernanda Monedeiro, Paweł Pomastowski, Maciej Milanowski, Tomasz Ligor and Bogusław Buszewski
Monitoring of Bactericidal Effects of Silver Nanoparticles Based on Protein Signatures and VOC Emissions from *Escherichia coli* and Selected Salivary Bacteria
Reprinted from: *J. Clin. Med.* **2019**, *8*, 2024, doi:10.3390/jcm8112024 73

Ildikó Judit Márton, József Horváth, Péter Lábiscsák, Bernadett Márkus, Balázs Dezső, Adrienn Szabó, Ildikó Tar, József Piffkó, Petra Jakus, József Barabás, Péter Barabás, Lajos Olasz, Zsanett Kövér, József Tőzsér, János Sándor, Éva Csősz, Beáta Scholtz and Csongor Kiss
Salivary IL-6 mRNA is a Robust Biomarker in Oral Squamous Cell Carcinoma
Reprinted from: *J. Clin. Med.* **2019**, *8*, 1958, doi:10.3390/jcm8111958 97

Óscar Rapado-González, Cristina Martínez-Reglero, Ángel Salgado-Barreira, Almudena Rodríguez-Fernández, Santiago Aguín-Losada, Luis León-Mateos, Laura Muinelo-Romay, Rafael López-López and María Mercedes Suarez-Cunqueiro
Association of Salivary Human Papillomavirus Infection and Oral and Oropharyngeal Cancer: A Meta-Analysis
Reprinted from: *J. Clin. Med.* **2020**, *9*, 1305, doi:10.3390/jcm9051305 . . . . **109**

Emanuela Martina, Anna Campanati, Federico Diotallevi and Annamaria Offidani
Saliva and Oral Diseases
Reprinted from: *J. Clin. Med.* **2020**, *9*, 466, doi:10.3390/jcm9020466 . . . . **127**

About the Editor

Pia Lopez-Jornet MD, DDS, PhD, University of Murcia (Spain): Full-time Professor of Oral Medicine at the University of Murcia; Director of the Master of Oral Medicine; Author of 120 publications indexed in the JCR, including 10 complete books and 9 book chapters; Dictator of numerous courses and conferences in national and international congresses; Head of the Consolidated Group at the Research Institute of Murcia (IMIB); A Participant of 10 clinical trials

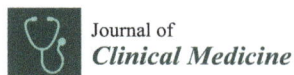
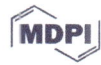

Editorial

Special Issue "Saliva and Oral Diseases"

Pia López Jornet

Oral Medicine in the Department of Stomatology, Faculty of Dentistry, University of Murcia, 30008 Murcia, Spain; majornet@um.es

Received: 16 June 2020; Accepted: 20 June 2020; Published: 23 June 2020

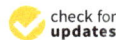

The discovery of microbial, immunological or molecular markers in saliva offers unique opportunities, and has caused our view of saliva to change drastically in recent years. Technological developments have made it possible to advance more rapidly and precisely in the diagnosis of diseases—opening a field of research with tremendous potential. In this special issue, The Journal of Clinical Medicine has gathered a panel of experts on saliva research. The different contributions cover a broad spectrum of topics, such as odontology, obesity, inflammation and cancer.

The possibility of monitoring, of seeing how and when a disease process starts and progresses, and of observing the outcomes of treatment based on noninvasive tools such as saliva, is a very desirable goal. One of the most ambitious aims of researchers is to detect salivary biomarkers and use them in clinical practice. Apart from the minimally invasive procedure involved in collecting saliva samples, we have the possibility of compiling lots of data and of exploring intraindividual variations—generating new challenges and opportunities.

In the area of oral diseases, Martina et al. [1] contributed a thorough review on the use of saliva from the perspective of the oral manifestations of skin disease, such as lichen planus, pemphigus, pemphigoid and psoriasis, and also addressed Sjögren's syndrome and oral cancer.

The working group of the University of Murcia, led by López–Jornet et al. [2], investigated burning mouth syndrome, contributing very interesting data on the determination of analytes in unstimulated saliva implicated in pain, stress and inflammation, and which can offer clues to help manage this complex chronic orofacial pain condition.

Regarding dental implantology, there is much controversy on the risks of peri-implantitis. Papi et al. [3] addressed this issue in an interesting study on saliva, examining the release of metals (titanium) in the development of peri-implantitis.

Overweight people/obesity is a worldwide social problem. Two interesting documents on this topic have been presented from different points of view: (a) Zalewska et al. [4] found overweight and obese adolescents to have an impaired systemic and salivary oxidative status when compared with adolescents of normal weight. (b) In a cross-sectional study, the Finnish research group of Syrjäläinen et al. [5] found that obese people may be susceptible to periodontal disease, though obesity was not associated to alterations in cytokines in saliva. In this regard, salivary cytokine alterations may be explained by a periodontal condition and smoking habit.

The use of saliva opens a range of possibilities for the management of patients with psoriasis. In this regard, biomarkers are explored that can be measured using simple, innocuous, painless and low-cost tests for use in clinical practice. The study [6] of variations in the concentration of TNF-α, IL-2, INF-γ, IL-10, nitric oxide, peroxynitrite, S-nitrosothiols and nitrotyrosine contributes to further our knowledge on the pathogenesis of psoriasis.

Studies on precise, profitable and noninvasive diagnostic methods require important efforts from all researchers. The emerging technologies developed in the last decade have contributed new value to the study of saliva.

Monedeiro et al. [7] used matrix-assisted laser desorption/ionization-time-of-flight mass spectrometry (MALDI-TOF MS) to investigate the influence of silver nanoparticles (AgNP) upon metabolism in bacterial strains. The approaches used may be useful for monitoring and assessing the response to treatment, based on the concentrations of AgNP.

In the field of oncology, we seek to identify molecular alterations and their relation to tumor progression, with a view of developing potential applications to diagnosis, prognosis and response to therapy. In this regard, the Hungarian group of Márton et al. [8] have analyzed the expression of IL-6 and mRNA in samples of saliva from patients with oral squamous cell carcinoma (OSCC), and recorded the differences with respect to the control group. On the other hand, the detection of human papillomavirus (HPV) from saliva (with or without oral rinses) represents a quick and easy noninvasive alternative for oral and oropharyngeal cancer screening in high-risk populations. Rapado–González et al. [9] conducted a meta-analysis providing additional evidence that salivary HPV is associated with oral and oropharyngeal cancer.

Lastly, it is important to create and integrate interdisciplinary research teams capable of advancing knowledge in the field of saliva, since we need to optimize identifying biomarkers and validate the findings in new patients, as well as establish targets for early therapeutic interventions.

Funding: This research received no external funding.

Conflicts of Interest: The authors declare no conflict of interest.

References

1. Martina, E.; Campanati, A.; Diotallevi, F.; Offidani, A. Saliva and Oral Diseases. *J. Clin. Med.* **2020**, *9*, 466. [CrossRef] [PubMed]
2. Lopez-Jornet, P.; Castillo Felipe, C.; Pardo-Marin, L.; Ceron, J.J.; Pons-Fuster, E.; Tvarijonaviciute, A. Salivary Biomarkers and Their Correlation with Pain and Stress in Patients with Burning Mouth Syndrome. *J. Clin. Med.* **2020**, *9*, 929. [CrossRef] [PubMed]
3. Papi, P.; Raco, A.; Pranno, N.; di Murro, B.; Passarelli, P.C.; D'Addona, A.; Pompa, G.; Barbieri, M. Salivary Levels of Titanium, Nickel, Vanadium, and Arsenic in Patients Treated with Dental Implants: A Case-Control Study. *J. Clin. Med.* **2020**, *9*, 1264. [CrossRef]
4. Zalewska, A.; Kossakowska, A.; Taranta-Janusz, K.; Zięba, S.; Fejfer, K.; Salamonowicz, M.; Kostecka-Sochoń, P.; Wasilewska, A.; Maciejczyk, M. Dysfunction of Salivary Glands, Disturbances in Salivary Antioxidants and Increased Oxidative Damage in Saliva of Overweight and Obese Adolescents. *J. Clin. Med.* **2020**, *9*, 548. [CrossRef] [PubMed]
5. Syrjäläinen, S.; Gursoy, U.K.; Gursoy, M.; Pussinen, P.; Pietiäinen, M.; Jula, A.; Salomaa, V.; Jousilahti, P.; Könönen, E. Salivary Cytokine Biomarker Concentrations in Relation to Obesity and Periodontitis. *J. Clin. Med.* **2019**, *8*, 2152. [CrossRef] [PubMed]
6. Monedeiro, F.; Pomastowski, P.; Milanowski, M.; Ligor, T.; Buszewski, B. Monitoring of Bactericidal Effects of Silver Nanoparticles Based on Protein Signatures and VOC Emissions from *Escherichia coli* and Selected Salivary Bacteria. *J. Clin. Med.* **2019**, *8*, 2024. [CrossRef] [PubMed]
7. Skutnik-Radziszewska, A.; Maciejczyk, M.; Flisiak, I.; Krahel, J.; Kołodziej, U.; Kotowska-Rodziewicz, A.; Klimiuk, A.; Zalewska, A. Enhanced Inflammation and Nitrosative Stress in the Saliva and Plasma of Patients with Plaque Psoriasis. *J. Clin. Med.* **2020**, *9*, 745. [CrossRef] [PubMed]
8. Márton, I.J.; Horváth, J.; Lábiscsák, P.; Márkus, B.; Dezső, B.; Szabó, A.; Tar, I.; Piffkó, J.; Jakus, P.; Barabás, J.; et al. Salivary IL-6 mRNA is a Robust Biomarker in Oral Squamous Cell Carcinoma. *J. Clin. Med.* **2019**, *8*, 1958.
9. Rapado-González, Ó.; Martínez-Reglero, C.; Salgado-Barreira, Á.; Rodríguez-Fernández, A.; Aguín-Losada, S.; León-Mateos, L.; Muinelo-Romay, L.; López-López, R.; Suarez-Cunqueiro, M.M. Association of Salivary Human Papillomavirus Infection and Oral and Oropharyngeal Cancer: A Meta-Analysis. *J. Clin. Med.* **2020**, *9*, 1305. [CrossRef] [PubMed]

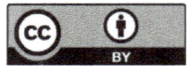

© 2020 by the author. Licensee MDPI, Basel, Switzerland. This article is an open access article distributed under the terms and conditions of the Creative Commons Attribution (CC BY) license (http://creativecommons.org/licenses/by/4.0/).

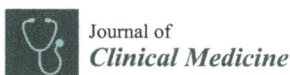

Article

Salivary Levels of Titanium, Nickel, Vanadium, and Arsenic in Patients Treated with Dental Implants: A Case-Control Study

Piero Papi [1], Andrea Raco [1], Nicola Pranno [1,*], Bianca Di Murro [1], Pier Carmine Passarelli [2], Antonio D'Addona [2], Giorgio Pompa [1,†] and Maurizio Barbieri [3,†]

1. Department of Oral and Maxillo-Facial Sciences, "Sapienza" University of Rome, 00161 Rome, Italy; piero.papi@uniroma1.it (P.P.); a.raco@hotmail.it (A.R.); bianca.dimurro@uniroma1.it (B.D.M.); giorgio.pompa@uniroma1.it (G.P.)
2. Division of Oral Surgery and Implantology, Department of Head and Neck, Oral Surgery, and Implantology Unit, Institute of Clinical Dentistry, Fondazione Policlinico Universitario A. Gemelli IRCCS-Università Cattolica del Sacro Cuore, 00168 Rome, Italy; piercarminepassarelli@hotmail.it (P.C.P.); antonio.daddona@policlinicogemelli.it (A.D.)
3. Department of Earth Sciences, "Sapienza" University of Rome, 00161 Rome, Italy; maurizio.barbieri@uniroma1.it
* Correspondence: nicola.pranno@uniroma1.it
† These two authors contributed equally.

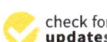

Received: 22 March 2020; Accepted: 23 April 2020; Published: 27 April 2020

Abstract: Background: Recent articles have hypothesized a possible correlation between dental implants dissolution products and peri-implantitis. The null hypothesis tested in this case-control study was that there would be no differences in salivary concentrations of titanium (Ti), vanadium (V), nickel (Ni) and arsenic (As) ions among patients with dental implants, healthy (Group A) or affected by peri-implantitis (Group B), compared to subjects without implants and/or metallic prosthetic restorations (Group C). Methods: Inductively coupled plasma mass spectrometry was used to analyze saliva samples. One-way repeated-measure analysis of variance (ANOVA) was used to identify statistically significant differences in the salivary level of Ti, V, Ni and As between the three groups. Results: A total of 100 patients were enrolled in the study (42 males and 58 females), distributed in three groups: 50 patients in Group C, 26 patients in Group B and 24 patients Group B. In our study, concentrations of metallic ions were higher in Group A and B, compared to the control group, with the exception of vanadium. However, there were no statistically significant differences ($p > 0.05$) for metallic ions concentrations between Group A and Group B. Conclusions: Based on our results, there are no differences in titanium or other metals concentrations in saliva of patients with healthy or diseased implants.

Keywords: dental implants; saliva; corrosion; titanium; metallic ions

1. Introduction

Dental implants are usually made of commercially pure titanium or titanium-based alloys (Ti-6Al-4V), these metals, as well as showing great long-term success and survival rates [1,2], are known to be bio compatibles and chemically inert in the oral cavity and consequently considered corrosion-resistant. Corrosion is a state of metal's deterioration caused by oxidation or chemical action, thwarted by a titanium dioxide layer (TiO_2), spontaneously covering the implant surface in presence of oxygen and providing great resistance and stability to the implant [3,4]. Nevertheless, titanium alloys can be affected by this gradual degradation and the structural and mechanical integrity of the implant may be jeopardized and at risk of failure. Corrosion leads to titanium dissolution, release and dispersion of metal ions and particles into soft and hard tissues either, which may be a possible factor in peri-implant inflammatory processes [5,6].

The factors that trigger corrosion are acidification of the oral environment or the release of lactic acid by bacteria, such as *Streptococcus mutans*, and also chemical stimuli by fluorides (with a concentration range greater than 100 ppm) normally present in home and professional oral care products [7–9].

Titanium and other metals particles released by dental implants are not totally bioinert: they induce the release of mediating inflammation cytokines, such as tumor necrosis factor-alpha (TNF-α), interleukin 1 beta (IL-1β) and the secretion of RANKL. These present an immunogenic potential which—by acting as a secondary inflammatory stimulus in peri-implantitis—amplifies bone resorption [10]

Under physiological conditions, osteoprotegerin (OPG) secreted by the fibroblasts of the periodontal ligament and osteoblasts, subtracts the receptor activator of nuclear factor kappa-B ligand (RANKL) from the link with its true receptor activator of nuclear factor kappa-B (RANK), creating a real competitive inhibition, preventing differentiation from the pre-osteoclast into osteoclasts and subsequent bone resorption [11,12]. In the presence of inflammation, an up-regulation of RANKL is associated with a down-regulation of OPG, which is produced in minimal quantities. The RANKL produced will, therefore, bind the RANK present on the osteoclastic precursors, with consequent massive bone resorption [13,14]

Furthermore, other kinds of corrosion can occur, such as mechanical corrosion due to functional stresses of implants or the cracking or weakening of its prosthetic components [7,8].

Once ultimately dispersed in the peri-implant environment, metal ions and particles are no longer biocompatible and inert, and are, therefore considered a potential incentive to the inflammatory process in peri-implantitis [5]. A study in mice immune cells has demonstrated that Titanium ions release pro-inflammatory cytokines involved in bone resorption, demonstrating that peri-implantitis may be directly related to corrosion and, therefore, with metal ions dispersion [15].

Peri-implantitis treatment and risk factors are still controversial [16,17], with incontrovertible evidence just for periodontitis, inadequate plaque control and lack of supportive periodontal therapy [18–20].

Furthermore, smoking, excess cement and other systemic conditions have all been described as potential risk indicators, however there is inconclusive evidence to draft clear conclusions [18,21–26].

Recent articles have hypothesized a possible correlation between titanium dissolution products and peri-implantitis [27–29] therefore, the aims of this case-control study were to evaluate salivary metallic ions dissolution in patients with dental implants, healthy or affected by peri-implantitis.

The null hypothesis tested was that there would be no differences in the salivary concentrations of titanium (Ti), vanadium (V), nickel (Ni) and arsenic (As) ions among patients with dental implants, healthy or affected by peri-implantitis, compared to subjects without implants and/or metallic prosthetic restorations.

2. Material and Methods

2.1. Study Design

To address the research purpose, the authors designed a case-control study, conducted at the Departments of Oral and Maxillo-Facial Sciences, at "Sapienza" University of Rome.

2.2. Study Population

From May 2018 to May 2019, all subjects who underwent previous implant surgery since January 2008 at the Oral Surgery Unit, Policlinico Umberto I, "Sapienza" University of Rome were identified and consecutively evaluated.

Each patient received detailed descriptions of the study protocol and all subjects signed an informed consent form to be included in the study population, according to the World Medical Declaration of Helsinki. The Institution Review Board of "Sapienza" approved the study (Ref. 4939/2018).

Eligible patients were divided into two groups: subjects with clinically healthy implants (Group A) and patients with peri-implantitis (Group B).

Patients in group A were enrolled in the study based on the following inclusion and exclusion criteria:

- Single crown implants functioning for >1 year
- No clinical signs of pathologies of the oral mucosa
- Age ≥ 18 years
- Implants classified as clinically healthy
- No antibiotic treatment in the previous three months
- Non-smoker
- No uncontrolled systemic diseases
- Not pregnant or breastfeeding
- No metal reconstruction, crowns or other prosthetic restorations present in the oral cavity

Patients in Group B had to meet the following inclusion and exclusion criteria:

- Single crown implants functioning for >1 year
- No clinical signs of pathologies of the oral mucosa
- Age ≥ 18 years
- Implants with a diagnosis of peri-implantitis
- No antibiotic treatment in the previous three months
- Non-smoker
- No uncontrolled systemic diseases
- Not pregnant or breastfeeding
- No metal reconstruction, crowns or other prosthetic restorations present in the oral cavity

Furthermore, a third group of patients (Group C) without dental implants, derived from a population of subjects attending the Oral Surgery Unit from May 2018 to May 2019 for wisdom tooth removal, was enrolled in accordance with the following inclusion and exclusion criteria:

- Absence of dental implants
- No metal reconstruction, crowns or other prosthetic restorations present in the oral cavity
- Age ≥ 18 years
- No clinical signs of pathologies of the oral mucosa
- No antibiotic treatment in the previous three months
- Non-smoker
- No uncontrolled systemic diseases
- Not pregnant or breastfeeding

2.3. Clinical Examination

Patients' data collected included sex and age.

For each implant, the following clinical measurements were recorded at six sites per implant by using a periodontal probe (PCP-Unc 15, Hu-Friedy®, Chicago, IL, USA):

- Probing pocket depth (PPD) measured in millimeters
- Plaque index (PI) recorded with dichotomic values (present/absent)
- Mucosal redness recorded with dichotomic values (present/absent)

- Suppuration recorded with dichotomic values (present/absent)
- Bleeding on probing recorded with dichotomic values (present/absent)

2.4. Radiographic Assessment

Mesial and distal implant crestal bone levels were measured on standardized (Rinn Centratore XCP Evolution 2003, Dentsply, Rome, Italy) digital periapical X-rays for each implant using a calibrated software (SOPRO Imaging, Acteon Group, Norwich, UK). The implant length and width were used as references for calibration of measurements, with the bone level digitally evaluated by measuring the distance between the implant shoulder and the first visible bone contact on the implant.

Case definitions for epidemiological or disease surveillance studies of the 2017 World Workshop on the Classification of Periodontal and Peri-Implant Diseases and Conditions were adopted to establish the diagnosis of peri-implant diseases [30].

2.5. Saliva Collection

Five milliliters of saliva were collected from each patient using the unstimulated drainage method, or alternatively by leaving the saliva flow passively from the lower lip directly into designated sterile tubes.

Patients were advised not to take food or drink and to avoid oral hygiene procedures before saliva collection.

All samples were stored at a temperature of 1 °C, in order to block any biologic process still in place.

2.6. ICP-MS Analysis

Samples were analyzed using a Thermo Scientific XSERIES2 ICP-MS instrument (Thermo-Fisher Scientific, Waltham, MA, USA) at the Department of Earth Sciences at "Sapienza" University of Rome. Samples were processed as previously described [29]. The concentrations of Ti, V, Ni and As were quantified in µg/L.

2.7. Statistical Analysis

The required sample size was calculated using statistics software (GPower 3.1.9.2, Heinrich-Heine-Universität, Düsseldorf, Germany). A power analysis using the repeated measures ANOVA with three measurements, an alpha level of 0.05 and a medium effect size ($f = 0.56$) showed that 100 subjects would be adequate to obtain 95% power in detecting a statistical difference in the salivary level of Ti, assuming a loss to follow-up of 20% [31].

A database was created using Excel (Microsoft, Redmond, WA, USA). Descriptive statistics were calculated for each variable. The Shapiro–Wilk test was used to determine whether or not the data conformed to a normal distribution.

One-way repeated-measures ANOVA was used to identify statistically significant differences in the salivary level of Ti, V, Ni and As between three different groups: Control group, patients with healthy implant and patients with implant affected by peri-implantitis. Pairwise Tukey honestly significant difference (HSD) test for multiple comparisons.

The chi-squared test of homogeneity was used to evaluate the presence of differences in the proportion of males and females among the three groups.

Data were evaluated using standard statistical analysis software (version 20.0, Statistical Package for the Social Sciences, IBM Corporation, Armonk, NY, USA). A p value <0.05 was considered as statistically significant.

3. Results

A total of 100 patients were enrolled in the study (42 males and 58 females; age 49.02 ± 11.37 years). The patients were thus distributed in the three groups: 50 patients in Group C, 26 patients in Group B and 24 patients Group B. There were no significant differences in the proportions of males and females in the three groups ($p = 0.620$). Patients' demographics are reported in Table 1.

Table 1. Sample demographic.

Study Variable	Group A	Group B	Group C
Sample size	26	24	50
Male	11	11	20
Female	15	13	30
Age (y) ± SD (range)	63.13 ± 17.72	70.52 ± 8.24	46.57 ± 9.23
Dental implants (n)	26	24	NA
Functional loading (y) ± SD (range)	7.8 ± 2.62	9.88 ± 3.52	NA
Mean PPD (mm)	3.2 ± 0.44	4.66 ± 1.32	NA
Mean MBL (mm)	0.89 ± 0.32	1.95 ± 1.43	NA

SD, standard deviation; PPD, probing pocket depth; MBL, marginal bone loss; NA, not applicable.

3.1. Titanium

The mean concentration of Ti was 136.65 ± 263.28 µg/L in the Group C, 489.60 ± 227.86 µg/L in the Group A and 492.83 ± 313.90 in the Group B. Statistical significant differences in mean concentration were found between the Group C and the Group A ($p < 0.001$) and between the Group C and the Group B ($p < 0.001$) (Table 2).

3.2. Nickel

The mean concentration of Ni was 4.77 ± 8.33 µg/L in the Group C, 24.99 ± 12.47 µg/L in the Group A and 23.50 ± 10.12 in the Group B. Statistical significant differences in mean concentration were found between the Group C and the Group A ($p < 0.001$) and between the Group C and Group B ($p < 0.001$) (Table 2).

3.3. Vanadium

The mean concentration of V was 1.30 ± 4.28 µg/L in the Group C, 2.27 ± 2.43 µg/L in the Group A and 2.01 ± 1.35 in the Group B. The group means of V concentration were not statistically significant different ($p = 0.440$) (Table 2).

3.4. Arsenic

The mean concentration of As was 0.01 ± 0.01 µg/L in the Group C, 2.20 ± 1.88 µg/L in the Group A and 1.54 ± 2.07 in the Group B. Statistical significant differences in mean concentration were found between the Group C and the Group A ($p < 0.001$) and between the Group C and the Group B ($p < 0.001$) (Table 2).

Table 2. Difference in the mean concentration of titanium, nickel vanadium and arsenic in the three groups.

Dependent Variable	(I) Groups	(J) Groups	Mean Difference (I-J)	Std. Error	Sig.	95% Confidence Interval	
						Lower Bound	Upper Bound
Titanium	Group C	Group A	−352.951280 *	59.517272	0.000	−494.61555	−211.28701
		Group B	−356.184613 *	61.127007	0.000	−501.68041	−210.68882
	Group A	Group C	352.951280 *	59.517272	0.000	211.28701	494.61555
		Group B	−3.233333	69.678791	0.999	−169.08426	162.61760
	Group B	Group C	356.184613 *	61.127007	0.000	210.68882	501.68041
		Group A	3.233333	69.678791	0.999	−162.61760	169.08426
Nickel	Group C	Group A	−20.215246 *	2.410887	0.000	−25.95369	−14.47680
		Group B	−18.728483 *	2.476093	0.000	−24.62213	−12.83483
	Group A	Group C	20.215246 *	2.410887	0.000	14.47680	25.95369
		Group B	1.486763	2.822503	0.858	−5.23142	8.20494
	Group B	Group C	18.728483 *	2.476093	0.000	12.83483	24.62213
		Group A	−1.486763	2.822503	0.858	−8.20494	5.23142
Vanadium	Group C	Group A	−0.965529	0.809320	0.460	−2.89189	0.96083
		Group B	−0.707260	0.831209	0.672	−2.68572	1.27120
	Group A	Group C	0.965529	0.809320	0.460	−0.96083	2.89189
		Group B	0.258269	0.947497	0.960	−1.99698	2.51352
	Group B	Group C	0.707260	0.831209	0.672	−1.27120	2.68572
		Group A	−0.258269	0.947497	0.960	−2.51352	1.99698
Arsenic	Group C	Group A	−2.193412 *	0.336286	0.000	−2.99385	−1.39298
		Group B	−1.525553 *	0.345382	0.000	−2.34764	−0.70347
	Group A	Group C	2.193412 *	0.336286	0.000	1.39298	2.99385
		Group B	0.667859	0.393701	0.212	−0.26924	1.60496
	Group B	Group C	1.525553 *	0.345382	0.000	0.70347	2.34764
		Group A	−0.667859	0.393701	0.212	−1.60496	0.26924

* The mean difference is significant at the 0.05 level. HSD, honestly significant difference.

4. Discussion

The aims of this study were to detect salivary metallic ions levels of Ti, V, Ni and As in patients with and without dental implants.

The metal concentration was measured by the use of ICP-MS, a versatile, rapid and extremely sensitive analytical technique used to determine different metallic and non-metallic inorganic substances present in concentrations lower than one part per billion.

Just a few studies have investigated the possible relationship of metallic ions dissolution and peri-implantitis, mainly focusing on titanium levels [27–29]

Safioti et al. first hypothesized a possible association between high titanium levels and implants affected by peri-implantitis, studying the metal concentration in submucosa plaque. The plaque samples were taken from the deepest points of the pockets of each implant through dental scalers (mini-five 1–2 Gracey) and then analyzed by ICP-MS. Results showed that implants with peri-implantitis had significantly ($p < 0.05$) higher titanium levels than healthy implants [27].

Olmedo et al. using the exfoliative cytology technique, measured the concentration of titanium particles in the peri-implant mucosa cells and found higher values in the group of patients affected by peri-implantitis compared to the group of patients with healthy implants [28,32].

In our study setting, attention was focused not only on titanium but also on other metals such as V, Ni and As.

Vanadium is ubiquitous: it is present in water and soil and its effects at systemic level are still debated: several authors have reported the use of vanadium in the treatment of diabetes mellitus, while others have correlated the long-term exposure with risk of cancer [33–36].

Nickel is known to be the cause of contact dermatitis and in general of allergic episodes, which can develop with serious consequences in the most sensitive subjects. Adverse reactions were documented in relation to orthodontic devices (brackets, arches) containing nickel. This element has a carcinogenic and mutagenic effects; therefore, exposure must be minimized [37–39].

Arsenic is one of the most widespread elements in nature: it can be found in soil, water, air and almost in all animal and plant tissues.

Arsenic poisoning can be acute (lethal) or chronic, caused by prolonged exposure even at low concentrations.

Martin-Camean et al. in 2014, in an in vivo study, evaluated the dissolution of different metal ions in the oral mucosa of subjects with orthodontic mini-implants. The epithelial cells of the oral mucosa were taken from each patient using a rubber brush. The samples were then analyzed through ICP-MS. The results reported only traces of vanadium, while the release of other elements occurred in the following growing order Cr < Ni < Ti < Cu < Al [40–42].

In our study, concentrations of metallic ions were higher in subjects with dental implants, either healthy or affected by peri-implantitis, compared to the control group, with the exception of vanadium.

Based on our results, metallic ions are detectable in the saliva of patients with dental implants; according to a recent systematic review conducted by Noronha Oliveira et al., degradation products—in the form of micro and nanoscale particles—can be found for different reasons, such as detachment from implant surface during surgical insertion, wear caused by micro-movements between contacting surfaces at implant connections, corrosive effects of therapeutic substances, like bleaching agents and fluorides or peri-implantitis treatment (mainly implantoplasty) [43].

In the present study, there were no statistically significant differences ($p > 0.05$) for metallic ions concentrations between patients with healthy dental implants and peri-implantitis subjects.

Our results are in contrast with the findings of Safioti et al. and Olmedo et al. [27,28]. However, in the above-mentioned articles, exclusion criteria did not limit enrollment to patients without other metallic prosthetic reconstructions and a control group without implants was not provided.

A recent systematic review by Gomes et al. [44] evaluated the diagnostic accuracy of biomarker levels in saliva to distinguish between healthy implants and implants affected by peri-implantitis. Based on their results, there was no clear evidence to support the use of salivary biomarkers (IL-6, IL-1β) in peri-implantitis detection. Pettersson et al. [45] performed gingival biopsies during surgical treatment of patients with severe periodontitis or peri-implantitis in order to evaluate titanium levels via ICP-MS. They found higher titanium values in peri-implantitis patients ($p < 0.001$) compared to periodontitis subjects, however samples were obtained after surgical treatment of dental implants and titanium release may be, therefore, exacerbated by ultrasonic scaling, as previously demonstrated by Eger et al. [46].

Furthermore, human samples from appropriate control groups (healthy implants and patients without metallic reconstructions) could not be obtained for ethical reasons.

Therefore, saliva collection and analysis through ICP-MS, as performed in the present study, seem a viable alternative to investigate data obtained by different populations.

5. Conclusions

Current evidence on the possible role of titanium or other metal particles in peri-implantitis pathogenesis is still controversial: in a recent critical review, Mombelli et al. concluded that there is poor specificity for the association of titanium particles and peri-implantitis, since metallic ions can be commonly detected in healthy and diseased peri-implant mucosa, as well as in gingiva of subjects without dental implants, being Tio2 used in multiple kinds of foods, toothpastes, cosmetics or medical pills [10].

Schwarz et al. in the latest World Workshop on the Classification of Periodontal and Peri-Implant Diseases and Conditions [18] stated that there was insufficient available evidence to consider titanium particles as a risk indicator for peri-implantitis.

Based on our results, concentrations of metallic ions were higher in subjects with dental implants, either healthy or affected by peri-implantitis, compared to the control group, with the exception of vanadium. No statistically significant differences were found in the metallic concentrations of healthy implants or peri-implantitis.

Future research should be orientated in conducting further studies, with a larger sample and a longitudinal design, to determine the role of titanium or other metals in peri-implantitis pathogenesis.

Author Contributions: P.P. and A.R. drafted the article, revised the paper and gave substantial contributions to the conception of the work; G.P. and A.D. gave substantial contributions to the conception of the work and revised the manuscript critically for important intellectual content. N.P. revised the paper, gave substantial contributions to the conception of the work and performed the statistical analysis. B.D.M. and P.C.P. revised the paper, gave substantial contributions to the conception of the work and recruited patients. M.B. gave substantial contributions to the conception of the work, revised the manuscript critically for important intellectual content and performed the ICP-MS analysis. All authors have read and agreed to the published version of the manuscript.

Conflicts of Interest: The authors declare they have no conflicts of interest related to this study.

References

1. De Angelis, F.; Papi, P.; Mencio, F.; Rosella, D.; Di Carlo, S.; Pompa, G. Implant survival and success rates in patients with risk factors: Results from a long-term retrospective study with a 10 to 18 years follow-up. *Eur. Rev. Med. Pharmacol. Sci.* **2017**, *21*, 433–437. [PubMed]
2. Rossi, F.; Lang, N.P.; Ricci, E.; Ferraioli, L.; Baldi, N.; Botticelli, D. Long-term follow-up of single crowns supported by short, moderately rough implants—A prospective 10-year cohort study. *Clin. Oral Implant. Res.* **2018**, *29*, 1212–1219. [CrossRef] [PubMed]
3. Li, J.; He, X.; Zhang, G.; Hang, R.; Huang, X.; Tang, B.; Zhang, X. Electrochemical corrosion, wear and cell behavior of ZrO(2)/TiO(2) alloyed layer on Ti-6Al-4V. *Bioelectrochemistry* **2018**, *121*, 105–114. [CrossRef]
4. Zhang, R.; Wan, Y.; Ai, X.; Liu, Z.; Zhang, D. Corrosion resistance and biological activity of TiO(2) implant coatings produced in oxygen-rich environments. *Proc. Inst. Mech. Eng. Part H* **2017**, *231*, 20–27. [CrossRef]
5. Delgado-Ruiz, R.; Romanos, G. Potential Causes of Titanium Particle and Ion Release in Implant Dentistry: A Systematic Review. *Int. J. Mol. Sci.* **2018**, *19*, 3585. [CrossRef] [PubMed]
6. Apaza-Bedoya, K.; Tarce, M.; Benfatti, C.A.M.; Henriques, B.; Mathew, M.T.; Teughels, W.; Souza, J.C.M. Synergistic interactions between corrosion and wear at titanium-based dentalimplant connections: A scoping review. *J. Periodontal Res.* **2017**, *52*, 946–954. [CrossRef] [PubMed]
7. Maruthamuthu, S.; Rajasekar, A.; Sathiyanarayanan, S.; Muthukumar, N.; Palaniswamy, N. Electrochemical behaviour of microbes on orthodontic wires. *Curr. Sci.* **2005**, *89*, 988–996.
8. Chang, J.C.; Oshida, Y.; Gregory, R.L.; Andres, C.J.; Barco, T.M.; Brown, D.T. Electrochemical study on microbiology-related corrosion of metallic dental materials. *Bio-Med. Mater. Eng.* **2003**, *13*, 281–295.
9. Souza, J.C.M.; Henriques, M.; Oliveira, R.; Teughels, W.; Celis, J.P.; Rocha, L.A. Do oral biofilms influence the wear and corrosion behavior of titanium titanium? *Biofouling* **2010**, *26*, 471–478. [CrossRef] [PubMed]
10. Mombelli, A.; Hashim, D.; Cionca, N. What is the impact of titanium particles and biocorrosion on implant survival and complications? A critical review. *Clin. Oral. Implant. Res.* **2018**, *29*, 37–53. [CrossRef]
11. Boyce, B.F.; Xing, L. Functions of RANKL/RANK/OPG in bone modeling and remodeling. *Arch. Biochem. Biophys.* **2008**, *473*, 139–146. [CrossRef] [PubMed]
12. Walsh, M.C.; Choi, Y. Biology of the RANKL-RANK-OPG System in Immunity, Bone, and Beyond. *Front. Immunol.* **2014**, *5*, 511.
13. Wachi, T.; Shuto, T.; Shinohara, Y.; Matono, Y.; Makihira, S. Release of titanium ions from an implant surface and their effect on cytokine production related to alveolar bone resorption. *Toxicology* **2015**, *327*, 1–9. [CrossRef] [PubMed]
14. Cadosch, D.; Al-Mushaiqri, M.S.; Gautschi, O.P.; Meagher, J.; Simmen, H.P.; Filgueira, L. Biocorrosion and uptake of titanium by human osteoclasts. *J. Biomed. Mater. Res.* **2010**, *95*, 1004–1010. [CrossRef] [PubMed]

15. Nishimura, K.; Kato, T.; Ito, T. Influence of titanium ions on cytokine levels of murine splenocytes stimulated with periodontopathic bacterial lipopolysaccharide. *Int. J. Oral. Maxillofac. Implant.* **2014**, *29*, 472–477.
16. La Monaca, G.; Pranno, N.; Annibali, S.; Cristalli, M.P.; Polimeni, A. Clinical and radiographic outcomes of a surgical reconstructive approach in the treatment of peri-implantitis lesions: A 5-year prospective case series. *Clin. Oral Implant. Res.* **2018**, *29*, 1025–1037. [CrossRef]
17. Mencio, F.; De Angelis, F.; Papi, P.; Rosella, D.; Pompa, G.; Di Carlo, S. A randomized clinical trial about presence of pathogenic microflora and risk of peri-implantitis: Comparison of two different types of implant-abutment connections. *Eur. Rev. Med. Pharmacol. Sci.* **2017**, *21*, 1443–1451.
18. Schwarz, F.; Derks, J.; Monje, A.; Wang, H.L. Peri-implantitis. *J. Periodontol.* **2018**, *89*, 267–290. [CrossRef]
19. Pimentel, S.P.; Shiota, R.; Cirano, F.R.; Casarin, R.C.V.; Pecorari, V.G.A.; Casati, M.Z.; Haas, A.N.; Ribeiro, F.V. Occurrence of peri-implant diseases and risk indicators at the patient and implant levels: A multilevel cross-sectional study. *J. Periodontol.* **2018**, *89*, 1091–1100. [CrossRef]
20. Dreyer, H.; Grischke, J.; Tiede, C.; Eberhard, J.; Schweitzer, A.; Toikkanen, S.E.; Glöckner, S.; Krause, G.; Stiesch, M. Epidemiology and risk factors of peri-implantitis: A systematic review. *J. Periodontal Res.* **2018**, *53*, 657–681. [CrossRef]
21. Papi, P.; Di Murro, B.; Pranno, N.; Bisogni, V.; Saracino, V.; Letizia, C.; Polimeni, A.; Pompa, G. Prevalence of peri-implant diseases among an Italian population of patients with metabolic syndrome: A cross-sectional study. *J. Periodontol.* **2019**, *90*, 1374–1382. [CrossRef]
22. Papi, P.; Letizia, C.; Pilloni, A.; Petramala, L.; Saracino, V.; Rosella, D.; Pompa, G. Peri-implant diseases and metabolic syndrome components: A systematic review. *Eur. Rev. Med. Pharmacol. Sci.* **2018**, *22*, 866–875. [PubMed]
23. Kotsakis, G.A.; Lan, C.X.; Barbosa, J.; Lill, K.; Chen, R.Q.; Rudney, J.; Aparicio, C. Antimicrobial agents used in the treatment of peri-implantitis alter the physicochemistry and cytocompatibility of titanium surfaces. *J. Periodontol.* **2016**, *87*, 809–819. [CrossRef] [PubMed]
24. Gurgel, B.C.V.; Montenegro, S.C.L.; Dantas, P.M.C.; Pascoal, A.L.B.; Lima, K.C.; Calderon, P.D.S. Frequency of peri-implant diseases and associated factors. *Clin. Oral Implant. Res.* **2017**, *28*, 1211–1217. [CrossRef] [PubMed]
25. Dalago, H.; Schuldt Filho, G.; Rodrigues, M.; Renvert, S.; Bianchini, M. Risk indicators for peri-implantitis: A cross-sectional study with 916 implants. *Clin. Oral Implant. Res.* **2017**, *28*, 144–150. [CrossRef] [PubMed]
26. Renvert, S.; Aghazadeh, A.; Hallström, H.; Persson, G.R. Factors related to peri-implantitis—A retrospective study. *Clin. Oral Implant. Res.* **2014**, *25*, 522–529. [CrossRef] [PubMed]
27. Safioti, L.M.; Kotsakis, G.A.; Pozhitkov, A.E.; Chung, W.O.; Daubert, D.M. Increased levels of dissolved titanium are associated with peri-implantitis—A cross-sectional study. *J. Periodontol.* **2017**, *88*, 436–442. [CrossRef]
28. Olmedo, D.G.; Nalli, G.; Verdú, S.; Paparella, M.L.; Cabrini, R.L. Exfoliative cytology and titanium dental implants: A pilot study. *J. Periodontol.* **2013**, *84*, 78–83. [CrossRef]
29. Barbieri, M.; Mencio, F.; Papi, P.; Rosella, D.; Di Carlo, S.; Valente, T.; Pompa, G. Corrosion behavior of dental implants immersed into human saliva: Preliminary results of an in vitro study. *Eur. Rev. Med. Pharmacol. Sci.* **2017**, *21*, 3543–3548.
30. Berglundh, T.; Armitage, G.; Araujo, M.G. Peri-implant diseases and conditions: Consensus report of workgroup 4 of the 2017 World Workshop on the Classification of Periodontal and Peri-Implant Diseases and Conditions. *J. Clin. Periodontol.* **2018**, *45*, 286–291. [CrossRef]
31. Faul, F.; Erdfelder, E.; Lang, A.G.; Buchner, A. G*Power 3: A flexible statistical power analysis program for the social, behavioral, and biomedical sciences. *Behav. Res. Methods* **2007**, *39*, 175–191. [CrossRef]
32. Olmedo, D.; Fernandez, M.M.; Guglielmotti, M.B.; Cabrini, R.L. Macrophages related to dental implant failure. *Implant Dent.* **2003**, *12*, 75–80. [CrossRef] [PubMed]
33. Zwolak, I. Vanadium carcinogenic, immunotoxic and neurotoxic effects: A review of in vitro studies. *Toxicol. Mech. Methods* **2014**, *24*, 1–12. [CrossRef] [PubMed]
34. Domingo, J.L.; Gómez, M. Vanadium compounds for the treatment of human diabetes mellitus: A scientific curiosity? A review of thirty years of research. *Food Chem. Toxicol.* **2016**, *95*, 137–141. [CrossRef] [PubMed]

35. Imtiaz, M.; Rizwan, M.S.; Xiong, S.; Li, H.; Ashraf, M.; Shahzad, S.M.; Shahzad, M.; Rizwan, M.; Tu, S. Vanadium, recent advancements and research prospects: A review. *Environ. Int.* **2015**, *80*, 79–88. [CrossRef] [PubMed]
36. Gruzewska, K.; Michno, A.; Pawelczyk, T.; Belarczyk, H. Essentiality and toxicity of vanadium supplements in health and pathology. *J. Physiol. Pharmacol.* **2014**, *65*, 603–611.
37. Lu, L.; Vollmer, J.; Moulon, C.; Weltzien, H.U.; Marrack, P.; Kappler, J. Components of the ligand for a Ni++ reactive human T cell clone. *J. Exp. Med.* **2003**, *197*, 567–574. [CrossRef]
38. Saito, M.; Arakaki, R.; Yamada, A.; Tsunematsu, T.; Kudo, Y.; Ishimaru, N. Molecular mechanisms of nickel allergy. *Int. J. Mol. Sci.* **2016**, *17*, 202. [CrossRef]
39. Girolomoni, G.; Gisondi, P.; Ottaviani, C.; Cavani, A. Immunoregulation of allergic contact dermtitis. *J. Dermatol.* **2004**, *31*, 264–270. [CrossRef]
40. Martín-Cameán, A.; Jos, A.; Calleja, A.; Gil, F.; Iglesias, A.; Solano, E.; Cameán, A.M. Validation of a method to quantify titanium, vanadium and zirconium in oral mucosa cells by inductively coupled plasma-mass spectrometry (ICP-MS). *Talanta* **2014**, *118*, 238–244. [CrossRef]
41. Martín-Cameán, A.; Jos, A.; Puerto, M.; Calleja, A.; Iglesias-Linares, A.; Solano, E.; Cameán, A.M. In vivo determination of aluminum, cobalt, chromium, copper, nickel, titanium and vanadium in oral mucosa cells from orthodontic patients with mini-implants by inductively coupled plasma-mass spectrometry (ICP-MS). *J. Trace Elem. Med. Biol.* **2015**, *32*, 13–20. [CrossRef] [PubMed]
42. Martín-Cameán, A.; Molina-Villalba, I.; Jos, A.; Iglesias-Linares, A.; Solano, E.; Cameán, A.M.; Gil, F. Biomonitorization of chromium, copper, iron, manganese and nickel in scalp hair from orthodontic patients by atomic absorption spectrometry. *Environ. Toxicol. Pharmacol.* **2014**, *37*, 759–771. [CrossRef] [PubMed]
43. Noronha Oliveira, M.; Schunemann, W.V.H.; Mathew, M.T.; Henriques, B.; Magini, R.S.; Teughels, W.; Souza, J.C.M. Can degradation products released from dental implants affect peri-implant tissues? *J. Periodontal Res.* **2018**, *53*, 1–11. [CrossRef] [PubMed]
44. Gomes, A.M.; Douglas-de-Oliveira, D.W.; Oliveira Costa, F. Could the biomarker levels in saliva help distinguish between healthy implants and implants with peri-implant disease? A systematic review. *Arch. Oral Biol.* **2018**, *96*, 216–222. [CrossRef]
45. Pettersson, M.; Pettersson, J.; Johansson, A.; Molin Thorén, M. Titanium release in peri-implantitis. *J. Oral Rehabil.* **2019**, *46*, 179–188. [CrossRef] [PubMed]
46. Eger, M.; Sterer, N.; Liron, T.; Kohavi, D.; Gabet, Y. Scaling of titanium implants entrains inflammation-induced osteolysis. *Sci. Rep.* **2017**, *7*, 39612. [CrossRef]

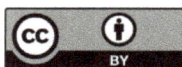

© 2020 by the authors. Licensee MDPI, Basel, Switzerland. This article is an open access article distributed under the terms and conditions of the Creative Commons Attribution (CC BY) license (http://creativecommons.org/licenses/by/4.0/).

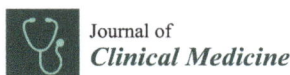

Article

Salivary Biomarkers and Their Correlation with Pain and Stress in Patients with Burning Mouth Syndrome

Pia Lopez-Jornet [1,*], Candela Castillo Felipe [2], Luis Pardo-Marin [3], Jose J. Ceron [3], Eduardo Pons-Fuster [4] and Asta Tvarijonaviciute [3]

1. Department Stomatology School of Medicine, Biomedical Research Institute (IMIB-Arrixaca), Faculty of Medicine and Odontology, University of Murcia, 30008 Adv Marques de los Velez s/n, Spain
2. Department Stomatology School of Medicine, Faculty of Medicine and Odontology, University of Murcia; 30008 Murcia, Span; candela.casti@gmail.com
3. Interdisciplinary Laboratory of Clinical Analysis, Interlab-UMU, Regional Campus of International Excellence 'Campus Mare Nostrum', University of Murcia, Espinardo, 30100 Murcia, Spain; lpm1@um.es (L.P.-M.); jjceron@um.es (J.J.C.); asta@um.es (A.T.)
4. Biomedical Research Institute (IMIB-Arrixaca), Faculty of Medicine and Odontology, University of Murcia, 30008 Murcia, Span; edupfl5@hotmail.com
* Correspondence: majornet@um.es; Tel.: +34-868-888-588

Received: 22 February 2020; Accepted: 25 March 2020; Published: 28 March 2020

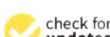

Abstract: Objective: To evaluate a panel of salivary analytes involving biomarkers of inflammation, stress, immune system and antioxidant status in patients with burning mouth syndrome (BMS) and to study their relationship with clinical variables. Materials and Methods: A total of 51 patients with BMS and 31 controls were consecutively enrolled in the study, with the recording of oral habits, the severity of pain using a visual analogue scale (VAS), the Hospital Anxiety and Depression (HAD) score and the Oral Health Impact Profile-14 (OHIP14) score. Resting whole saliva was collected with the drainage technique, followed by the measurement of 11 biomarkers. Results: The salivary flow was higher in patients with BMS. Among all the biomarkers studied, significantly higher levels of alpha-amylase, immunoglobulin A (IgA), and macrophage inflammatory protein-4 (MIP4) and lower levels of uric acid and ferric reducing activity of plasma (FRAP) were observed in the saliva of patients with BMS as compared to the controls ($p < 0.05$ in all cases). Positive correlations were found between pain, oral quality of life and anxiety scores and salivary biomarkers. Conclusions: BMS is associated with changes in salivary biomarkers of inflammation, oxidative stress and stress, being related to the degree of pain and anxiety.

Keywords: saliva; IgA; alpha-amylase; uric acid; stress; inflammation

1. Introduction

The International Association for the Study of Pain (IASP) defines burning mouth syndrome (BMS) as an intraoral burning or dysesthetic sensation that manifests daily for more than two hours over three months, with no evidence of clinical lesions [1]. The epidemiological data on BMS are largely contradictory, in part because of a lack of strict compliance with the diagnostic criteria of the disorder. Nevertheless, BMS is estimated to affect 4% of the general population and 18–33% of all postmenopausal women [2–6]. The symptoms are generally focused on the tongue and lips and are almost always bilateral. The palate and other locations within the oral cavity are less commonly affected. Although much has been published about BMS, its underlying etiopathogenesis is largely unknown, and complex interactions among local, systemic and psychogenic factors are believed to be involved [2,7,8]. For these reasons, BMS is poorly diagnosed, and in many cases management is deficient, a situation that causes frustration for both physicians and patients [3,5]. In the same way as with other chronic pain syndromes, BMS is characterized by associated psychological problems. Changes in personality and mood state, particularly anxiety and depression, are a typical finding in patients with BMS [2,9].

The use of saliva as a sample for clinical analysis has increased in recent decades. Saliva is a body fluid that reflects the physiological condition of the body. It can be easily collected using non-invasive and relatively inexpensive methods [4,5], and it is gaining attention as a source of biomarkers in different oral and systemic pathologies [10]. In BMS an increase in amylase (a marker of the adrenergic system) and immunoglobulin A (IgA) (a marker of the immune system) have been found [11–14]. However, to the authors' knowledge, there have been no studies in which a panel of analytes reflecting possible pathogenic and psychological factors were evaluated in this disease, and also compared with the degree of stress and pain.

The objective of this study was to evaluate how a panel of biomarkers of inflammation represented by complement C4 (CC4), α1-antitrypsin (a1AT), C-reactive protein (CRP), macrophage inflammatory protein-4 (MIP4), pigment epithelium-derived factor (PEDF), serum amyloid P (SAP), haptoglobin (Hp), a panel of biomarkers of oxidative stress integrated by uric acid and ferric reducing activity of plasma (FRAP), the salivary alpha-amylase (sAA) as a marker of the adrenergic system and total immunoglobulin A (IgA) as a marker of the innate immune system can be altered in patients with BMS, and study their possible relation with the degree of pain and stress of the patients was measured by visual analogue scale (VAS) and the Hospital Anxiety and Depression (HAD) score. Also, the possible influence of oral health was evaluated.

2. Material and Methods

2.1. Study Design and Subjects

A cross-sectional study was carried out with data compiled between January 2018 and September 2019 in the Dental Clinic of the University of Murcia (Murcia, Spain). All the patients were informed about the study and gave consent to participation in the trial, which was approved by the local Clinical Research Ethics Committee (Ref.: 2203/2018). The following inclusion criteria were established: patients over 18 years of age with a diagnosis of BMS based on exhaustive oral examination, laboratory findings and the patient profile and symptoms [15], presenting continuous symptoms of oral burning or pain persisting for at least two hours per day, lasting longer than three months, without paroxysms and not following any unilateral nerve trajectory, and with no clinical mucosal alterations. The patients underwent blood testing to confirm the absence of alterations (including blood count, glucose, serum iron, ferritin and transferrin, folic acid and vitamin B12 levels). Cancer patients and individuals with known liver or kidney disease were excluded, as were those with oral diseases other than BMS such as Sjögren's syndrome or ongoing infection, thyroid diseases, coagulation disorders, psychiatric disease, and pregnant or nursing women.

The healthy controls were recruited from the Dental School of the University of Murcia and consisted of patients with the same sociosanitary characteristics and matched for age and gender. Following the procurement of written informed consent, a structured questionnaire was administered to confirm the absence of significant medical conditions. The study was carried out following the STROBE (Strengthening the Reporting of Observational studies in Epidemiology) guidelines.

In all cases, patients were not included in the study if their samples showed hemolysis as determined by visual inspection [16,17].

2.2. Data Collection

A structured interview was used to collect sociodemographic and clinical information as well as data referring to smoking and alcohol consumption. The patients were evaluated by a trained professional (C.C.F.) who conducted the interviews and explorations, administered the questionnaires and collected the saliva samples.

An extraoral and intraoral exploration was carried out, documenting the presence of caries and missing teeth. Pain intensity was scored using a visual analogue scale (VAS) (0 = no pain and 10 = worst possible pain) [18].

The Hospital Anxiety and Depression (HAD) scale [19] was used to assess the emotional state of the participants. This instrument consists of two subscales relating to anxiety (HAD-A) and depression (HAD-D). Concerning the interpretation of the HAD scale, scores of > 10 indicate the probable presence of anxiety or depression, scores of ≤ 7 indicate no significant anxiety or depression, and scores of 8–10 are of borderline significance.

The evaluation of the oral quality of life, in turn, was based on the Oral Health Impact Profile-14 (OHIP14) score [20].

2.3. Saliva Collection

Resting whole saliva was collected using a standardized method [18]. To avoid possible contamination from other sources, the patients were instructed to rinse the mouth thoroughly before saliva sample collection. The subjects were required to avoid heavy physical exercise one hour before sampling. Unstimulated saliva was obtained using the draining method for 5 min. The samples were collected at about the same time in all subjects (8:00 to 11:00 a.m.). The saliva was vortexed and centrifuged (3000× g for 10 min at 4 °C) immediately after collection, and the supernatant was transferred into polypropylene tubes and stored at −80 °C until analysis.

2.4. Biochemical Analysis

Complement C4, a1AT, CRP, MIP4, PEDF and SAP in saliva were analyzed using a commercially available kit (Human Neurodegenerative Disease Magnetic Bead Panel 2, Neuroscience Multiplex Assay; Life Science, Darmstadt, Germany) according to the manufacturer's instructions. Values were calculated based on a standard curve constructed for the assay. Saliva total protein quantification was done using a commercially available colorimetric kit for measuring urine and low-complexity region (LCR) proteins (protein in urine and CSF, Spinreact, Barcelona, Spain) and validated for human saliva [21]. Uric acid was measured using a colorimetric commercial kit (Uric acid, Beckman Coulter Inc., Fullerton, CA, USA) following the International Federation of Clinical Chemistry and Laboratory Medicine (IFCC) method [21]. Total IgA was evaluated with a commercial ELISA kit (Bethyl, Montgomery, TX, USA) previously validated for use with human saliva samples [18]. FRAP (ferric reducing ability of plasma) measurement was based on the method described by Benzie and Strain [22] with some modifications [23]. Hp levels were measured in saliva using a homemade immunoassay as previously described [24]. Salivary alpha-amylase (sAA) activity was measured using a colorimetric commercial kit (Alpha-Amylase, Beckman Coulter Inc., Fullerton, CA, USA) following the IFCC method as previously reported and validated [25].

2.5. Statistical Analysis

For the descriptive statistical analysis of the sample, the basic descriptive methods were used, with calculation of the frequencies, mean, median, standard deviation (SD) and 25th and 75th percentile values. The comparison of means between groups was based on the Student's t-test or Mann–Whitney test, depending on the data distribution as verified with the Kolmogorov–Smirnov test, and the homogeneity of groups was confirmed. Clinical scores, smoking and alcohol consumption habits, as well as sex distribution among the two groups, were explored using the chi-square test. The correlations between variables were checked using the partial correlation corrected by age and sex. Previous studies that also analyzed biomarkers in saliva in patients with burning mouth syndrome, such as sAA and total IgA, have been able to detect differences with 30 or fewer individuals in each group considering $\alpha = 0.05$ and $\beta = 0.20$ [11]. Based on these data we assumed that the study was sufficiently powered ($n_{controls} = 31$; $n_{BMS} = 51$) to achieve our aims. Differences and associations among groups were considered statistically significant when $p < 0.05$.

3. Results

The study sample consisted of 82 consecutively enrolled individuals (71 females and 11 males), of which 51 were diagnosed with BMS while the remaining 31 constituted the control group. Table 1 describes the characteristics of each group. Statistically significant differences were not detected in sex, age or smoking and alcohol consumption habits between the two groups of patients ($p > 0.05$).

Table 1. General characteristics of participants.

Variable	Controls	SBA	p
Sex, n (%)			0.083 [c]
Women	26 (76.5)	45 (88.2)	
Men	5 (14.7)	6 (11.8)	
Age, mean (SD) years	58.3 (11.05)	59.12 (12.29)	0.765 [a]
Smoking, n (%)			0.292 [c]
Yes	10 (32.3)	11 (21.6)	
No	18 (58.1)	29 (56.9)	
Former smoker	3 (9.7)	11 (21.6)	
Alcohol consumption, n (%)			0.212 [c]
Less than once a week	21 (61.8)	31 (60.8)	
Daily	2 (5.9)	9 (17.6)	
Weekends only	11 (32.4)	11 (21.6)	
Tooth brushing, n (%)			0.236 [c]
No	0 (0)	1 (2)	
Less than once a day	1 (3.2)	1 (2)	
Once a day	7 (22.6)	5 (9.8)	
Twice a day	14 (45.2)	18 (35.3)	
≥3 times a day	9 (29)	26 (51)	
Dental floss, n (%)			**0.006** [c]
No	23 (74.2)	22 (43.1)	
Yes	8 (25.8)	29 (56.9)	
Mouthwashes, n (%)			0.080 [c]
No	28 (90.3)	38 (74.5)	
Yes	3 (9.7)	13 (25.5)	
Missing teeth, mean (SD)	2.1 (2.82)	5.8 (8.3)	**0.004** [b]
Missing teeth groups, n (%)			0.098 [c]
1–5	29 (93.5)	39 (76.5)	
6–9	0 (0)	5 (9.8)	
<10	2 (6.5)	7 (13.7)	

Table 1. *Cont.*

Variable	Controls	SBA	p
Caries, mean (SD)	0.42 (0.99)	0.2 (1.13)	0.121 [b]
OHIP14, mean (SD)	14.33 (1.37)	33.1 (9.02)	**<0.001** [b]
HAD-A, mean (SD)	3.77 (2.3)	8.71 (3.82)	**<0.001** [b]
HAD-D, mean (SD)	2.9 (2.4)	4.1 (3.6)	0.292 [b]
VAS, mean (SD)	0 (0)	8.12 (1.77)	**<0.001** [b]
VAS groups, n (%)			
Mild		1 (2.0)	
Moderate		16 (31.4)	
Severe		34 (66.7)	

a, Student's t-test; b, Mann–Whitney test; c, Pearson's chi-square. Bold type denotes statistical significance.

Concerning oral hygiene and health, the controls and patients with BMS did not present statistically significant differences in habits related to tooth brushing and use of mouthwashes, while patients with BMS used more dental floss than controls ($p < 0.01$). In turn, controls presented a comparatively greater number of caries, though the difference was not statistically significant ($p > 0.05$), and significantly fewer missing teeth compared with the BMS group ($p < 0.01$).

Of the clinical variables, the mean burning sensation score in patients with BMS was greater than 8, while it was equal to 0 in healthy controls. The OHIP14 score was 2.3-fold higher in the BMS group as compared with the control group ($p = 0.001$).

Concerning the psychological profile as evaluated by the HAD scale, the anxiety scores among the patients were 2.3-fold higher than in controls ($p < 0.001$). While HAD-D, although being 1.4-fold higher in patients, did not show statistically significant differences between the two groups ($p > 0.05$).

Resting whole saliva flow was 1.4-fold greater in the BMS group as compared to healthy controls ($p < 0.05$) (Figure 1a and Table S1). The study of biomarkers in resting whole saliva yielded significant differences between the cases (patients with BMS) and controls for sAA ($p < 0.01$) and IgA ($p < 0.05$) (Figure 1a,b and Table S1).

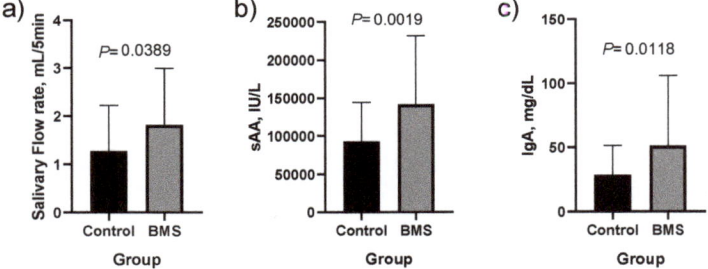

Figure 1. Salivary flow rate (**a**), salivary alpha-amylase (sAA; (**b**)) and immunoglobulin A (IgA; (**c**)) in healthy controls ($n = 31$) and patients with burning mouth syndrome (BMS; $n = 51$). Differences of medians and means±SD for salivary flow are 0.54 and 0.75 ± 0.41, for sAA they are 48,660 and 109,536 ± 41,492 and for IgA they are 22.47 and 34.01 ± 12.72.

When absolute values of salivary biomarkers were corrected by salivary flow, sAA, IgA and MIP4 showed statistically higher concentrations in patients with BMS as compared with healthy controls (Figure 2 and Table S1). When values were corrected by total protein content, statistically significantly higher levels in patients with BMS were observed for sAA and lower for uric acid and FRAP (Figure 3 and Table S1).

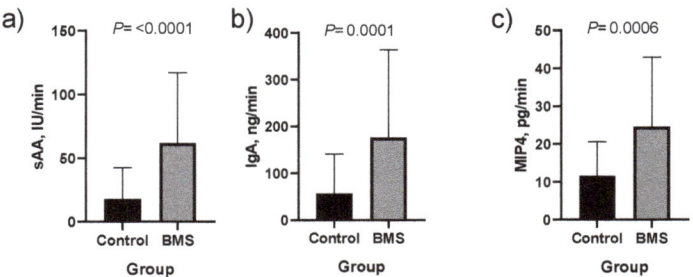

Figure 2. Salivary alpha-amylase (sAA; (**a**)), immunoglobulin A (IgA; (**b**)) and macrophage inflammatory protein-4 (MIP4; (**c**)) corrected by salivary flow in healthy controls ($n = 31$) and patients with burning mouth syndrome (BMS; $n = 51$). Difference of medians and means ± SD for sAA are 44.0 and 47.4 ± 15.91, for IgA are 119.9 and 147.6 ± 38.4 and for MIP4 are 13.0 and 33.6 ± 27.2.

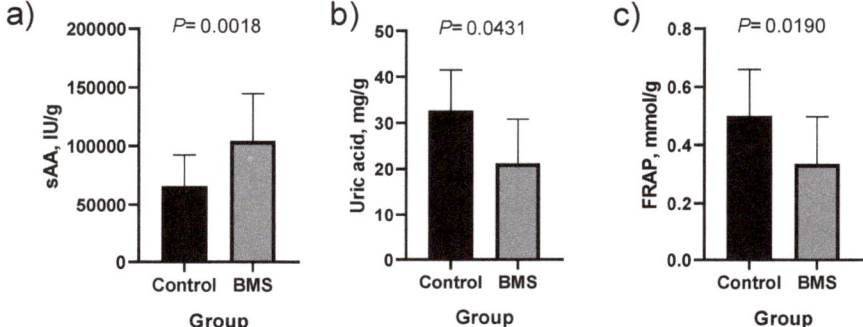

Figure 3. Salivary alpha amylase [sAA; (**a**)], uric acid (**b**) and ferric reducing activity [FRAP; (**c**)] corrected by salivary total protein content in healthy controls ($n = 31$) and patients with burning mouth syndrome (BMS; $n = 51$). Difference of medians and means ± SD for sAA are 38,525 and 33,653 ± 15,365, for uric acid are −11.5 and −7585 ± 4593 and for FRAP are −0.17 and −0.1413 ± 0.06614.

Partial correlation data are given in Table S2. When absolute values were evaluated, a positive correlation was detected between VAS and total proteins ($r = 0.241$; $p < 0.05$), sAA ($r = 0.260$; $p < 0.05$) and IgA ($r = 0.334$; $p < 0.01$); HAD-A was correlated with total proteins ($r = 0.251$; $p < 0.05$), IgA ($r = 0.302$; $p < 0.05$), PEDF ($r = 0.351$; $p < 0.01$) and MIP4 ($r = 0.267$; $p < 0.05$) and HAD-D with IgA ($r = 0.261$; $p < 0.05$), PEDF ($r = 0.363$; $p < 0.01$) and MIP4 ($r = 0.271$; $p < 0.05$); OHIP14 was correlated with IgA ($r = 0.273$; $p < 0.05$).

After data were corrected by salivary flow, statistically significant correlations remained between VAS and sAA ($r = 0.269$; $p < 0.05$) and IgA ($r = 0.367$; $p < 0.01$); between HAD-A and IgA ($r = 0.338$; $p < 0.01$), PEDF ($r = 0.297$; $p < 0.05$) and MIP4 ($r = 0.264$; $p < 0.05$); between HAD-D and PEDF ($r = 0.386$; $p = 0.01$) and MIP4 ($r = 0.269$; $p < 0.05$) and between OHIP14 and IgA ($r = 0.313$; $p < 0.01$).

After data were corrected by salivary flow, negative correlations appeared between sAA and OHIP14 ($r = -0.242$; $p < 0.05$) and between HAD-A and FRAP ($r = 0.250$; $p < 0.05$) and CRP ($r = -0.243$; $p < 0.05$).

4. Discussion

Burning mouth syndrome is a clinically relevant form of chronic orofacial pain [1–3]. The diagnosis of the syndrome remains a challenge for health professionals due to the discrepancy between the intensity of pain as reported by the patient and the absence of objective clinical lesions. In this study we therefore focused on the identification of potential biomarkers capable of reflecting the physiopathological changes involving pain, psychological stress and inflammation that occur in the context of the disease. Of 11 biomarkers evaluated in the present study, three—sAA, IgA and MIP4—were found to be increased, and two—uric acid and FRAP—were found to be decreased in the saliva of patients with BMS versus controls, suggesting that these patients can present with alterations in immune response, pro-inflammatory status and oxidative stress that are related to pain sensation and psychological stress.

In the present study, a higher salivary flow rate was detected in patients with BMS as compared with healthy controls. In the scientific literature, controversy exists regarding this topic since some authors did not detect changes in salivary flow between controls and patients with BMS [12–14], while others observed lower flow rates in patients with BMS [9,11,26]. Similarly, different authors reported divergent results related to total protein content in the saliva of patients with BMS, as some of them detected decreased [27], increased [12,14] or unchanged (present study) salivary total protein content in these patients when compared with controls. The characteristics of the method or device used to collect the samples and the analytical assays used may have influenced the results obtained and, therefore, the differences among the different studies. It is therefore important to follow the same guidelines for sample collection and processing to enable comparison of the results from different studies.

Since components present in saliva have different origins, i.e., are locally secreted by salivary glands or oral mucosa, or pass from blood among other, and can be affected by non-uniform salivary flow rate, the need to correct values of salivary biomarker by flow rate, total protein content or salivary osmolarity versus use of their absolute value is being increasingly acknowledged and studied by different authors [25,28]. In this study we aimed to evaluate the results without any adjustment, and we also corrected salivary flow or total protein content to gain knowledge about the possible effect that these corrections can have in this particular disease. When levels of biomarkers without any adjustment by saliva flow or protein content were compared between healthy and diseased patients, statistically significant changes were detected only in sAA and IgA. Correction by salivary flow rate allowed identification of the increased levels of MIP4 in the saliva of patients with BMS but also yielded higher differences between the studied groups for IgA in accordance with previously reported data [29]. When values were corrected by total protein content the presence of oxidative stress in patients with BMS was detected, as levels of uric acid and FRAP were lower compared to controls. Therefore, in BMS, correcting salivary values by flow rate and total protein content would be recommended in this disease since it can detect additional changes in salivary analytes that are correlated with the clinical condition of the patient.

sAA is considered to be a sensitive biomarker of stress-related changes that reflect the activity of the sympathetic nervous system (SNS) [30]. Most patients with BMS experience chronic pain and have a poorer quality of life than do healthy individuals [9]. Furthermore, chronic pain characterizing BMS was associated with psychological problems, specifically personality and mood changes, anxiety and depression. The results of this study agree with these findings and previous reports that detected higher sAA levels in the saliva of patients with BMS [12,14] since patients included in the present study showed both higher anxiety scores and sAA levels; however, another study did not detect changes in sAA between healthy controls and patients with BMS, and differences in the severity of the disease in the population evaluated or in the assay used could be the cause of these differences [9]. A weak positive correlation between sAA (expressed in absolute concentrations and when corrected by flow) and burning sensation was detected, which could indicate that increases in this enzyme could be influenced in part by pain.

Salivary IgA was another biomarker that showed statistically significant differences among controls and patients in the studied population, being higher in patients with BMS. These data are consistent with those reported by other authors [12–14]. Furthermore, a higher difference between the two groups was detected when IgA was corrected by salivary flow resulting in an increase of 1.8-fold to 2.9-fold change between the two groups. IgA is an immune glycoprotein that acts as a defense against pathogens [31]. Nevertheless, different studies have suggested that changes in salivary IgA can also be associated with stress [32]. This hypothesis would be supported by the observed positive correlations between IgA in saliva and oral quality of life, burning sensation and anxiety in the studied population. In addition, MIP, a biomarker of the innate immune system [33], was also increased in patients with BMS and weakly positively correlated with anxiety and depression scores, suggesting that the immune system is implicated in the pathogenesis of BMS.

In the present study, when the results were corrected by protein content, patients with BMS had lower salivary FRAP and uric acid, suggesting the presence of oxidative stress, and in the case of FRAP, it was weakly correlated with HAD-A, which would indicate that this increase could be influenced by stress. The two markers are closely related since uric acid was the main component (up to 60%) of the FRAP assay [22]. Uric acid is considered to be the most important antioxidant molecule in saliva since it is responsible for approximately 70% of the total antioxidant capacity of this body fluid. As a reactive oxygen species scavenger, it helps stabilize arterial pressure and oxidative stress [21,34–36]. In turn, alterations in its levels in saliva were associated with acute stress [34] and different local and systemic pathologies such as oral lichen planus [37] or nephropathies [38]. Previous studies that evaluated salivary uric acid in patients with BMS did not find statistically significant changes as compared with healthy controls [16,20], although these studies did not make corrections for total protein content.

A limitation of the study is the fact that the measurements were limited to a single time-point. Variations of these markers in the same individual should be investigated in the context of future studies with a larger sample size to increase the power, and by employing multiple samplings over time, resulting in more accurate estimations. Furthermore, it would be of interest to apply the biomarkers that showed significant changes in a larger population to corroborate the results of this study. Finally, the possible blood contamination in saliva samples should have been evaluated using more sensitive methods, such as determination of hemoglobin or transferrin, although these methods were shown to be affected by different factors such as age, hormones and salivary flow among others [16]. Conversely, visual inspection was shown to be sufficient in the case of determining some of the analytes including oxidative stress markers in saliva without interfering with the results [17].

5. Conclusions

In conclusion, patients with BMS showed changes in biomarkers associated with stress such as sAA and IgA, with the immune system such as MIP4 and oxidative stress such as uric acid and FRAP in saliva as compared with healthy controls, which are related to clinical variables including burning sensation and anxiety. Moreover, in this particular disease, the study of the absolute values but also the values corrected by flow and total protein would be recommended. Overall, biomarkers that were shown to change differently between groups could potentially help clinicians not only with diagnosis but also in objectively evaluating the severity of this disease, although further large-scale studies should first be performed to collaborate our findings.

Supplementary Materials: The following are available online at http://www.mdpi.com/2077-0383/9/4/929/s1: Table S1: Median and interquartile range data of salivary markers in healthy controls (n = 31) and patients suffering from BMS (n = 51); Table S2: Partial correlation adjusted for age and sex.

Author Contributions: Conceptualization, P.L.-J., C.C.F. and A.T.; Methodology, P.L.-J., C.C.F. and A.T.; Software, L.P.-M., J.J.C. and A.T.; Validation, P.L.-J., C.C.F and E.P.-F.; Formal Analysis, P.L.-J., A.T., L.P.-M. and J.J.C.; Investigation, P.L.-J., C.C.F., L.P.-M. and A.T.; Resources, P.L.-J., C.C.F., J.J.C. and A.T.; Data Curation, P.L.-J. and C.C.F.; Writing-Original, P.L.-J., J.J.C. and A.T.; Draft Preparation, E.P.-F.; Writing-Review & Editing, P.L.-J., A.T. and J.J.C.; Supervision, All authors; Project Administration, P.L.-J. and A.T. All authors have read and agreed to the published version of the manuscript.

Funding: A.T. has a post-doctoral fellowshisp "Ramón y Cajal" supported by the "Ministerio de Economía y Competitividad", Spain. This work was supported by a grant from the Program for Research Groups of Excellence of the Seneca Foundation, Murcia, Spain (grant 19894/GERM/15).

Conflicts of Interest: The authors declare no conflict of interest.

References

1. Scala, A.; Checchi, L.; Montevecchi, M.; Marini, I.; Giamberardino, M.A. Update on burning mouth syndrome: Overview and patient management. *Crit. Rev. Oral Biol. Med.* **2003**, *14*, 275–291. [CrossRef]
2. Olesen, J. Headache classification committee of the International Headache Society (IHS) the international classification of headache disorders, 3rd edition. *Cephalalgia* **2018**, *38*, 1–211.
3. Kohorst, J.J.; Bruce, A.J.; Torgerson, R.R.; Schenck, L.A.; Davis, M.D.P. The prevalence of burning mouth syndrome: A population-based study. *Br. J. Dermatol.* **2015**, *172*, 1654–1656. [CrossRef] [PubMed]
4. Klasser, G.D.; Fischer, D.J.; Epstein, J.B. Burning mouth syndrome: Recognition, understanding, and management. *Oral Maxillofac. Surg. Clin. N. Am.* **2008**, *20*, 255–271. [CrossRef] [PubMed]
5. López-Jornet, P.; Camacho-Alonso, F.; Andujar-Mateos, P.; Sánchez-Siles, M.; Gómez-García, F. Burning mouth syndrome: Update. *Med. Oral Patol. Oral Cir. Bucal* **2010**, *15*, e562-8. [CrossRef] [PubMed]
6. Ariyawardana, A.; Chmieliauskaite, M.; Farag, A.M.; Albuquerque, R.; Forssell, H.; Nasri-Heir, C.; Klasser, G.D.; Sardella, A.; Mignogna, M.D.; Ingram, M.; et al. World Workshop on Oral Medicine VII: Burning mouth syndrome: A systematic review of disease definitions and diagnostic criteria utilized in randomized clinical trials. *Oral Dis.* **2019**, *25*, 141–156. [CrossRef] [PubMed]
7. Jääskeläinen, S.K. Is burning mouth syndrome a neuropathic pain condition? *Pain* **2018**, *159*, 610–613. [CrossRef]
8. Ritchie, A.; Kramer, J.M. Recent advances in the etiology and treatment of burning mouth syndrome. *J. Dent. Res.* **2018**, *97*, 1193–1199. [CrossRef]
9. Kim, H.-I.; Kim, Y.-Y.; Chang, J.-Y.; Ko, J.-Y.; Kho, H.-S. Salivary cortisol, 17β-estradiol, progesterone, dehydroepiandrosterone, and α-amylase in patients with burning mouth syndrome. *Oral Dis.* **2012**, *18*, 613–620. [CrossRef]
10. Tvarijonaviciute, A.; Martinez-Subiela, S.; Lopez-Jornet, P.; Lamy, E. *Saliva in Health and Disease: The Present and Future of a Unique*; Springer: Berlin/Heidelberg, Germany, 2020; ISBN 9783030376802.
11. Imura, H.; Shimada, M.; Yamazaki, Y.; Sugimoto, K. Characteristic changes of saliva and taste in burning mouth syndrome patients. *J. Oral Pathol. Med.* **2016**, *45*, 231–236. [CrossRef]
12. Nagler, R.M.; Hershkovich, O. Sialochemical and gustatory analysis in patients with oral sensory complaints. *J. Pain* **2004**, *5*, 56–63. [CrossRef] [PubMed]
13. Granot, M.; Nagler, R.M. Association between regional idiopathic neuropathy and salivary involvement as the possible mechanism for oral sensory complaints. *J. Pain* **2005**, *6*, 581–587. [CrossRef] [PubMed]
14. Hershkovich, O.; Nagler, R.M. Biochemical analysis of saliva and taste acuity evaluation in patients with burning mouth syndrome, xerostomia and/or gustatory disturbances. *Arch. Oral Biol.* **2004**, *49*, 515–522. [CrossRef] [PubMed]
15. Silvestre, F.J.; Silvestre Rangil, J.; López Jornet, P. Burning mouth syndrome: A review and update. *Rev. Neurol.* **2015**, *60*, 463.
16. Kang, J.H.; Kho, H.S. Blood contamination in salivary diagnostics: Current methods and their limitations. *Clin. Chem. Lab. Med.* **2018**, *57*, 1115–1124. [CrossRef]
17. Kamodyová, N.; Baňasová, L.; Janšáková, K.; Koborová, I.; Tóthová, L'.; Stanko, P.; Celec, P. Blood contamination in Saliva: Impact on the measurement of salivary oxidative stress markers. *Dis. Markers* **2015**, *2015*, 479251. [CrossRef]
18. Lopez-Jornet, P.; Cayuela, C.A.; Tvarijonaviciute, A.; Parra-Perez, F.; Escribano, D.; Ceron, J. Oral lichen planus: Salival biomarkers cortisol, immunoglobulin A, adiponectin. *J. Oral Pathol. Med.* **2016**, *45*, 211–217. [CrossRef]
19. Zigmond, A.S.; Snaith, R.P. The hospital anxiety and depression scale. *Acta Psychiatr. Scand.* **1983**, *67*, 361–370. [CrossRef]
20. Montero-Martin, J.; Bravo-Pérez, M.; Albaladejo-Martínez, A.; Hernández-Martin, L.A.; Rosel-Gallardo, E.M. Validation the Oral Health Impact Profile (OHIP-14sp) for adults in Spain. *Med. Oral Patol. Oral Cir. Bucal* **2009**, *14*, 14.
21. González-Hernández, J.M.; Franco, L.; Colomer-Poveda, D.; Martinez-Subiela, S.; Cugat, R.; Cerón, J.J.; Márquez, G.; Martínez-Aranda, L.M.; Jimenez-Reyes, P.; Tvarijonaviciute, A. Influence of sampling conditions, salivary flow, and total protein content in uric acid measurements in Saliva. *Antioxidants* **2019**, *8*, 389. [CrossRef]

22. Benzie, I.F.F.; Strain, J.J. The Ferric Reducing Ability of Plasma (FRAP) as a measure of "Antioxidant Power": The FRAP assay. *Anal. Biochem.* **1996**, *239*, 70–76. [CrossRef] [PubMed]
23. Tvarijonaviciute, A.; Aznar-Cayuela, C.; Rubio, C.P.; Ceron, J.J.; López-Jornet, P. Evaluation of salivary oxidate stress biomarkers, nitric oxide and C-reactive protein in patients with oral lichen planus and burning mouth syndrome. *J. Oral Pathol. Med.* **2017**, *46*, 387–392. [CrossRef] [PubMed]
24. Tvarijonaviciute, A.; Zamora, C.; Ceron, J.J.; Bravo-Cantero, A.F.; Pardo-Marin, L.; Valverde, S.; Lopez-Jornet, P. Salivary biomarkers in Alzheimer's disease. *Clin. Oral Investig.* **2020**. [CrossRef] [PubMed]
25. Contreras-Aguilar, M.D.; Escribano, D.; Martínez-Subiela, S.; Martínez-Miró, S.; Rubio, M.; Tvarijonaviciute, A.; Tecles, F.; Cerón, J.J. Influence of the way of reporting alpha-amylase values in saliva in different naturalistic situations: A pilot study. *PLoS ONE* **2017**, *12*, e0180100. [CrossRef]
26. Lee, Y.C.; Hong, I.K.; Na, S.Y.; Eun, Y.G. Evaluation of salivary function in patients with burning mouth syndrome. *Oral Dis.* **2015**, *21*, 308–313. [CrossRef]
27. Tammiala-Salonen, T.; Söderling, E. Protein composition, adhesion, and agglutination properties of saliva in burning mouth syndrome. *Eur. J. Oral Sci.* **1993**, *101*, 215–218. [CrossRef]
28. Lindsay, A.; Costello, J.T. Realising the potential of urine and saliva as diagnostic tools in sport and exercise medicine. *Sport. Med.* **2016**, *47*, 1–21. [CrossRef]
29. Marcotte, H.; Lavoie, M.C. Oral microbial ecology and the role of salivary Immunoglobulin A. *Microbiol. Mol. Biol. Rev.* **1998**, *62*, 71–109. [CrossRef]
30. Ngamchuea, K.; Chaisiwamongkhol, K.; Batchelor-Mcauley, C.; Compton, R.G. Chemical analysis in saliva and the search for salivary biomarkers-a tutorial review. *Analyst* **2018**, *143*, 81–99. [CrossRef]
31. Yoo, E.M.; Morrison, S.L. IgA: An immune glycoprotein. *Clin. Immunol.* **2005**, *116*, 3–10. [CrossRef]
32. Yang, Y.; Koh, D.; Ng, V.; Lee, C.Y.; Chan, G.; Dong, F.; Goh, S.H.; Anantharaman, V.; Chia, S.E. Self perceived work related stress and the relation with salivary IgA and lysozyme among emergency department nurses. *Occup. Environ. Med.* **2002**, *59*, 836–841. [CrossRef] [PubMed]
33. De Nadaï, P.; Chenivesse, C.; Gilet, J.; Porte, H.; Vorng, H.; Chang, Y.; Walls, A.F.; Wallaert, B.; Tonnel, A.B.; Tsicopoulos, A.; et al. CCR5 usage by CCL5 induces a selective leukocyte recruitment in human skin xenografts In vivo. *J. Investig. Dermatol.* **2006**, *126*, 2057–2064. [CrossRef] [PubMed]
34. Goodman, A.M.; Wheelock, M.D.; Harnett, N.G.; Mrug, S.; Granger, D.A.; Knight, D.C. The hippocampal response to psychosocial stress varies with salivary uric acid level. *Neuroscience* **2016**, *339*, 396–401. [CrossRef] [PubMed]
35. Albert, U.; De Cori, D.; Aguglia, A.; Barbaro, F.; Bogetto, F.; Maina, G. Increased uric acid levels in bipolar disorder subjects during different phases of illness. *J. Affect. Disord.* **2015**, *173*, 170–175. [CrossRef]
36. Wen, S.; Cheng, M.; Wang, H.; Yue, J.; Wang, H.; Li, G.; Zheng, L.; Zhong, Z.; Peng, F. Serum uric acid levels and the clinical characteristics of depression. *Clin. Biochem.* **2012**, *45*, 49–53. [CrossRef]
37. Bakhtiari, S.; Toosi, P.; Samadi, S.; Bakhshi, M. Assessment of uric acid level in the saliva of patients with oral lichen planus. *Med. Princ. Pract.* **2017**, *26*, 57–60. [CrossRef]
38. Bilancio, G.; Cavallo, P.; Lombardi, C.; Guarino, E.; Cozza, V.; Giordano, F.; Palladino, G.; Cirillo, M. Saliva for assessing creatinine, uric acid, and potassium in nephropathic patients. *BMC Nephrol.* **2019**, *20*, 242. [CrossRef]

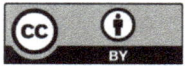

© 2020 by the authors. Licensee MDPI, Basel, Switzerland. This article is an open access article distributed under the terms and conditions of the Creative Commons Attribution (CC BY) license (http://creativecommons.org/licenses/by/4.0/).

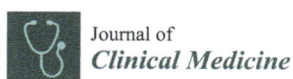
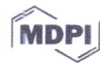

Article

Enhanced Inflammation and Nitrosative Stress in the Saliva and Plasma of Patients with Plaque Psoriasis

Anna Skutnik-Radziszewska [1], Mateusz Maciejczyk [2], Iwona Flisiak [3], Julita Krahel [3], Urszula Kołodziej [4], Anna Kotowska-Rodziewicz [4], Anna Klimiuk [5] and Anna Zalewska [5,*]

1. Experimental Dentistry Laboratory, Medical University of Bialystok, 1 Jana Kilinskiego Street, 15-089 Bialystok, Poland; anna.skutnik@o2.pl
2. Department of Hygiene, Epidemiology and Ergonomics, Medical University of Bialystok, 2c Mickiewicza Street, 15-022 Bialystok, Poland; mat.maciejczyk@gmail.com
3. Department of Dermatology and Venereology, Medical University of Bialystok, 14 Zurawia Street 15-540 Bialystok, Poland; iwona.flisiak@umb.edu.pl (I.F.); julita.leonczuk@gmail.com (J.K.)
4. Department of Restorative Dentistry, Medical University of Bialystok, 24A M. Sklodowskiej-Curie Street, 15-276 Bialystok, Poland; ulakol@poczta.onet.pl (U.K.); kotowskanna@wp.pl (A.K-R.)
5. Experimental Dentistry Laboratory, Medical University of Bialystok, 24A M. Sklodowskiej-Curie Street, 15-276 Bialystok, Poland; annak04@poczta.onet.pl
* Correspondence: azalewska426@gmail.com

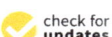

Received: 10 February 2020; Accepted: 9 March 2020; Published: 10 March 2020

Abstract: Psoriasis is the most common inflammatory skin disease, characterized by the release of proinflammatory cytokines from lymphocytes, keratinocytes, and dendritic cells. Although psoriasis is considered an immune-mediated inflammatory disease, its effect on secretory activity of salivary glands and quantitative composition of saliva is still unknown. The aim of this study was to evaluate the secretion of saliva as well as several selected inflammation and nitrosative stress biomarkers in unstimulated and stimulated saliva as well as plasma of psoriasis patients. We demonstrated that, with progressing severity and duration of the disease, the secretory function of the parotid and submandibular salivary glands is lost, which is manifested as decreased unstimulated and stimulated saliva secretion and reduced salivary amylase activity and total protein concentration. The levels of tumor necrosis factor-alpha (TNF-α), interleukin-2 (IL-2), and interferon-gamma (INF-γ) were significantly higher, whereas interleukin-10 (IL-10) content was considerably lower in unstimulated and stimulated saliva of patients with psoriasis compared to the controls, and the changes increased with the disease duration. Similarly, we observed that the intensity of nitrosative stress in the salivary glands of psoriasis patients depended on the duration of the disease. By means of receiver operating characteristic (ROC) analysis, we showed that the evaluation of nitric oxide (NO), nitrotyrosine, and IL-2 concentration in non-stimulated saliva with high sensitivity and specificity differentiated psoriasis patients on the basis of the rate of saliva secretion (normal salivation vs. hyposalivation). In summary, the dysfunction of salivary glands in psoriasis patients is caused by inflammation and nitrosative stress.

Keywords: plaque psoriasis; salivary glands; saliva; cytokines; nitrosative stress

1. Introduction

Psoriasis vulgaris is a skin inflammatory disease, the third most common among autoimmune diseases [1]. The pathogenesis of psoriasis involves the combination of genetic susceptibility, aberrant immune response, and several environmental factors (injuries, viral infections, medications taken, food intolerances). Typical features of psoriasis vulgaris include an immune-mediated process in which the key role is played by Th1 cells (T-helper 1). The presence of antigen-specific CD4+ (dendritic cell) T cells secreting type 1 cytokines: interferon-gamma (INF-γ), interleukin-2 (IL-2), and tumor necrosis factor-alpha (TNF-α) was observed in psoriatic skin lesions [2,3]. Moreover, the imbalance between Th1 and Th2 cells in psoriasis was confirmed by studies that showed interleukin-10 (IL-10) deficiency in psoriatic skin lesions [4]. Recent findings suggest that redox imbalance in the blood and skin of patients with psoriasis, resulting from the immune system stimulation, plays as important role in the pathogenesis of plaque psoriasis as the inflammatory process itself. It has been shown that, in the course of psoriasis, oxidative stress (OS) is primarily caused by reduced activity/concentration of antioxidants [5–9] and leads to increased oxidative modification of cellular elements of skin and plasma [6,10,11]. Plasma and erythrocyte product of lipid peroxidation (malondialdehyde, MDA) is considered a biomarker of plaque psoriasis exacerbation [12,13].

The detrimental inflammatory milieu and increased production of free radicals (ROS) associated with plaque psoriasis are not limited to the skin, but are also responsible for the growing number of comorbidities, including cardiological diseases, metabolic syndrome, chronic kidney disease, mood disorders, and salivary gland diseases [5,14–17].

Saliva produced by salivary glands performs numerous important functions in the oral cavity: hydrating it, removing harmful waste products and bacteria, participating in the remineralization of dental hard tissues, maintaining redox balance, and being involved in immune responses [18–20]. Disorders of both the composition and amount of saliva secreted into the oral cavity have physiological and psychological consequences. Therefore, it is very important to understand the mechanisms leading to salivary gland dysfunction in the course of systemic diseases. Unfortunately, the pathophysiology of salivary gland disorders in psoriasis is still unknown. In our previous work, we demonstrated that plaque psoriasis is accompanied by salivary redox imbalances with the prevalence of oxidation reactions. We observed that redox equilibrium in the submandibular glands was more vulnerable, and antioxidant capacity of the submandibular glands decreased with the disease duration [15]. There have been very few studies on the modification of saliva inflammatory components in psoriatic patients. Ganzetti et al. [21] demonstrated higher levels of TNF-α, transforming growth factor-beta (TGF-β), and interleukin-1 (IL-1β) in the saliva of psoriatic subjects vs. the controls. Unfortunately, most patients with psoriasis had also been diagnosed with periodontitis or gingivitis. Consequently, the observed cytokine changes in saliva reflected periodontal inflammation and not psoriasis-related salivary changes, and thus they did not explain the pathophysiology of salivary gland dysfunctions in the course of this disease. It has been evidenced that pro-inflammatory cytokines boost the expression of the inducible nitric oxide (NO) synthase (*i*NOS) in the cells, which results in increased NO synthesis in inflamed joints [22]. It was proven that NO and other reactive nitrogen intermediates affect a vast number of physiological functions of salivary glands, including exocytosis, water secretion, salivary blood flow, and non-specific immunological reactions [23–25]. The contribution of nitrosative stress to the pathophysiology of salivary glands in the course of psoriasis is unknown.

An ideal biomarker is characterized by simple determination as well as high sensitivity, specificity, and repeatability. It should also enable the identification of the patient's physiological and pathological status and response to the applied treatment [26]. Numerous biomarkers have been suggested for easier diagnosis of psoriasis and monitoring of its treatment. However, studies on psoriasis biomarkers have been based on blood tests, examining skin fragments, conducting genetic tests, and transcriptomics. The results of these studies were divergent, and therefore neither was considered reliable nor was accepted as a psoriasis marker [27]. Saliva is a mixture of secretions of large salivary glands and gingival fluid. It also contains almost all the elements present in the blood and passing through the spaces between cells as part of an inter- and paracellular transport. It is also relatively easy and safe to collect, providing a new, non-invasive way to diagnose numerous general diseases [28–32].

Thus, the aim of this work was to explore the mechanisms responsible for salivary gland dysfunction in psoriasis. We compared the concentrations of TNF-α, IL-2, INF-γ, IL-10, NO, peroxynitrite, S-nitrosothiols, and nitrotyrosine in the saliva and blood of psoriatic subjects with hyposalivation and normal salivation vs. healthy controls. The goal of our study was also to search for salivary biomarkers to assess the severity of psoriasis and the accompanying salivary complications.

2. Materials and Methods

We obtained the consent of the Local Research Ethics Committee in Bialystok (permission number: R-I-002/563/2018). All patients as well as healthy subjects were informed about the purpose of the study and its risks and benefits, and they all consented to the collection of saliva and blood samples.

This experiment included psoriatic patients applying for treatment to the Department of Dermatology and Venereology of the Medical University of Bialystok. The reason for reporting to the hospital was exacerbation of psoriasis symptoms. Patients had not undergone general treatment of psoriasis within 2 preceding years. The only acceptable forms of treatment included local application of ointment with glucocorticosteroids, but not during 3 preceding months. The severity of skin lesions was assessed using the previously described Psoriasis Area and Severity Index (PASI) [15].

A total of 60 healthy patients participated in the study, who were individuals reporting for check-up visits to the Department of Restorative Dentistry at the Medical University of Bialystok, and were matched to the group of patients in terms of age and sex.

Within 6 preceding months, participants did not take any medicines that could affect the composition and secretion of saliva, as well as vitamins, antioxidants, and antibiotics. The participants from the control group were generally healthy, and patients with psoriasis did not have any accompanying diseases. The inclusion criteria was absence of periodontal pathology (periodontal pocket depth (PPD) < 2 mm, did not bleed during the probing) and no inflammatory or fungal changes on the oral mucosa. Only subjects without acrylic dentures were included in the study. The patients as well as healthy controls were not addicted to alcohol and did not smoke cigarettes.

One of the criteria differentiating the dysfunction of salivary glands is reduced flow of unstimulated saliva (NWS) [18]. Therefore, to delineate the influence of psoriasis vulgaris on the parotid and submandibular glands, psoriatic patients were divided into two groups: with reduced NWS (psoriasis hyposalivation-PH, $n = 30$) and normal NWS (psoriasis normal secretion- PN, $n = 30$). The limit value for NWS was assumed at ≤ 0.2 mL/min, which is considered the minimum value of NWS for healthy population [18]. Moreover, the minimum value of NWS in our control group was 0.21 mL/min.

The number of patients was confirmed by the test as sufficient, and the test power was 0.9. Clinical characteristics of the patients are presented in Table 1.

Table 1. Clinical characteristics of plaque psoriasis patients and control subjects.

Patient Characteristics		Control $n = 60$	PN $n = 30$	PH $n = 30$
Sex	Male n (%)	23 (38.33%)	13 (43.33%)	10 (33.33%)
	Female n (%)	37 (61.67%)	17 (56.67%)	20 (66.67%)
Age (years)		52 ± 5	49 ± 6	51 ± 3
Height (cm)		172 ± 6	176 ± 3	169 ± 8
Weight (kg)		75 ± 1	72 ± 3	74 ± 1
Duration of psoriasis (years)		ND	9.7 ± 3.4	18.52 ± 7.8
PASI		ND	10.39 ± 2.4	18.29 ± 4.6
Psoriasis in the family	<1 n (%)	ND	18 (60%)	6 (20%)
	≥1 n (%)	ND	12 (40%)	24 (80%)

Table 1. Cont.

Patient Characteristics	Control n = 60	PN n = 30	PH n = 30
Blood Tests			
RBC ($10^6/\mu L$)	4.54 ± 0.54	4.23 ± 0.65	4.89 ± 0.87
HCT (%)	40.25 ± 6.5	42.45 ± 4.25	45.21 ± 0.89
PLT ($10^3/\mu L$)	275 ± 56	245 ± 87	292 ± 23
WBC ($10^3/\mu L$)	6.5 ± 2.2	7.05 ± 1.8	6.98 ± 1.86
CRP (mg/L)	1.5 ± 0.5	8.56 ± 6.3	6.32 ± 7.56
Glc (mg/dL)	69 ± 9.8	72 ± 9.8	75 ± 6.5
ALT (U/L)	27.56 ± 12.3	24.36 ± 9.68	27.24 ± 6.35
AST (U/L)	28.54 ± 12.25	30.23 ± 6.52	28.98 ± 8.64
Dental Characteristics			
DMFT	20 ± 3	19 ± 6	21 ± 2
GI	0.2 ± 0.1	0.2 ± 0.2	0.1 ± 0.2
PPD	1.5 ± 0.5	1.0 ± 0.5	1.0 ± 0.5
Dental implants	0	0	0

Abbreviations: ALT—alanine transferase; AST—aspartate transaminase; CRP—C-reactive protein; DMFT—decayed, missing, filled teeth index; GI—gingival index; Glc—D-glucose; HCT—hematocrit; n—number of patients; PASI—Psoriasis Area and Severity Index; PBI—papilla bleeding index; PLT—platelets; RBC—red blood cells; WBC—white blood cells. ND-not defined.

2.1. Blood Collection

Blood was collected at fasting, either at the admission of a patient to the hospital or during routine tests in case of control subjects. Blood was collected at 5 mL using an S-Monovette EDTA K3 tube (Sarstedt, Nümbrecht, Germany). The samples were then centrifuged (3000 × g, 10 min, 4 °C). No hemolysis was observed in any of the obtained plasma samples. To prevent sample oxidation, 0.5 M Butylated hydroxytoluene BHT (Sigma-Aldrich, Saint Louis, MO, USA; 10 µL/mL blood) was added [28]. Plasma was frozen (−82 °C). The samples were stored deep-frozen for no longer than 6 months.

2.2. Saliva Collection

The examined material was unstimulated and stimulated (SWS) total saliva collected from the patient by the spitting method [28]. Saliva was collected in the morning, on an empty stomach, between 8 a.m. and 10 a.m. in order to minimize the effect of daily changes on saliva secretion. The participants had refrained from taking any drugs for 8 hours prior to the examination. Saliva was collected in a separate room, in a sitting position with the head slightly inclined downwards, with minimized face and lip movements, and after a 5-minute adaptation period. Next, the patient rinsed the mouth three times with water at room temperature. The saliva collected during the first minute was discarded. The subsequent batches of saliva (the patient actively spat out the saliva accumulated in the bottom of the oral cavity) were collected into a plastic centrifuge tube placed in an ice container. NWS was collected for 15 minutes, and SWS was collected after a 5-minute break. Stimulation was performed by dropping 100 µL of 2% citric acid on the tip of the tongue every 20 seconds, for 5 minutes. To prevent sample oxidation, 0.5 M BHT (Sigma-Aldrich, Saint Louis, MO, USA; 10 µL/mL blood) was added to the saliva [33]. The volume of each sample was measured with a pipette calibrated to 0.1 mL. Saliva secretion was calculated by dividing the volume of the obtained saliva by the number of minutes of its collection. The collected saliva was centrifuged (20 minutes, 4 °C, 10,000 × g) [33]. The sediments were discarded, and supernatant fluid was divided into portions of 200 µL each, frozen in −80 °C, and stored until assayed, but for no longer than 6 months.

2.3. Stomatological Examination

After saliva collection, stomatological examinations were performed by one dentist (A.S.-R.), in artificial light, using a dental mirror, probe, and periodontal probe (Hossa International, Warsaw, Poland; design and construction in accordance with WHO guidelines) according to WHO criteria [34]. The dental status of each participant was assessed on the basis of the DMFT index (decayed, missing, filled teeth). The condition of periodontal tissues was assessed using GI (gingival index) and probing pocket depth (PPD) were assessed at teeth 16, 21, 24, 36, 41, and 44. The PPD and occurrence of bleeding were assessed after gently introducing the probe into the gingival space parallel to the long axis of the tooth, to the depth of perceived resistance posed by the bottom of the gingival gap. Four surfaces of each examined tooth (mesial, distal, buccal, and lingual) were examined. In the case of GI, we used a scale of 0 to 3. The sum of the values, from four surfaces divided by 4, determined the level of the PPD/ gingival index for a given tooth. Then, the results were added and divided by the number of teeth examined. In 25 participants, the inter-rater agreement between the examiner (A.S.-R.) and other experienced dentists (U.K., A.K.) was performed. The reliability for DMFT was $r = 0.99$, for GI was $r = 0.89$, and for PPD was $r = 0.94$. If bleeding during probing or PPD deeper than 2 mm were found, previously collected saliva was discarded and the patient was excluded from the study. Thus, 53 patients with psoriasis and 37 healthy controls who had bleeding of probing and/or PPD > 2 mm were disqualified from the study.

2.4. Biochemical Assays

All determinations of plasma, NWS, and SWS were performed in duplicate samples. The absorbance/fluorescence was measured using an Infinite M200 PRO Multimode Microplate Reader (Tecan Group Ltd., Männedorf, Switzerland). The results were standardized to 1 mg of protein.

2.5. Pro-Inflammatory Cytokines

The concentrations of TNF-α, IL-2, IL-10, and INF-γ were determined by the ELISA method using commercial kits from EIAab Science Inc. Wuhan (Wuhan, China), according to the manufacturer's instructions.

2.6. Nitrosative Stress

The concentration of NO was determined spectrophotometrically using the Griess reagent—a solution of sulfanilic acid and α-naphthylamine in acetic acid [35]. The reaction of nitrates with sulfanilamide produces N-(1-naphthyl)-ethylenediamine dihydrochloride, the absorbance of which was measured at 490 nm wavelength.

The concentration of S-nitrosothiols was determined spectrophotometrically on the basis of the reaction of the Griess reagent with Cu^{2+} copper ions [36]. The solution was shaken and set aside for 20 minutes, and then the absorbance was measured at 490 nm [37].

Peroxynitrite concentration was determined spectrophotometrically via a test using peroxynitrite decomposition followed by nitration of 4-hydroxyphenylacetic acid (4-HPA) and glycyltyrosine [38]. The reaction resulted in the production of nitrophenol, the absorbance of which was measured at 320 nm wavelength.

The concentration of nitrotyrosine was determined by ELISA using the Nitrotyrosine ELISA kit from Immunodiagnostik AG (Bensheim, Germany), following the manufacturer's instructions provided in the package.

2.7. Salivary Protein

Salivary protein content was determined using the bicinchoninic acid (BCA) method (Pierce BCA Protein Assay; Thermo Scientific (Rockford, IL, USA)). Bovine serum albumin was used as a standard.

2.8. Salivary Amylase

The activity of salivary amylase (EC 3.2.1.1.) was determined colorimetrically using 3,5-dinitrosalicylic acid (DNS) as a substrate [39]. By this method, starch was transformed by amylase to maltose, and was measured at 540 nm by the complex with DNS.

2.9. Statistical Analysis

The obtained results were assessed statistically by means of one-way analysis of variance (ANOVA). The significance of differences between individual groups was determined with the post-hoc Tukey's HSD test, and normal distribution was confirmed via the Shapiro–Wilk test. The correlations between the examined parameters were described using the Pearson correlation coefficient. The value of $p < 0.05$ was considered statistically significant. In order to assess the diagnostic usefulness between plaque psoriasis patients with normal salivary secretion and hyposalivation, receiver operating characteristic (ROC) curves were generated and then the area under the curve (AUC) was calculated. Every parameter had its optimal limit values determined, which simultaneously provided high sensitivity and specificity. The analysis of the data was performed in the statistical program GraphPad Prism 8.3.0 for MacOS.

3. Results

3.1. Inflammatory Cytokines

3.1.1. NWS

The concentration of IL-2 (↑10.91%, $p = 0.007$; ↑33.64%, $p < 0.0001$, respectively) and INF-γ (↑33.11%, $p \leq 0.0001$; ↑57.34%, $p \leq 0.0001$, respectively) in NWS of psoriasis patients with normal and decreased saliva secretion was significantly higher than in the control group. Moreover, concentrations of IL-2 (↑20.50%, $p \leq 0.0001$) and INF-γ (↑18.21%, $p = 0.005$) in NWS of patients with hyposalivation were considerably higher than in psoriasis patients with normal saliva secretion. TNF-α concentration in the NWS of psoriasis patients with hyposalivation was significantly higher than in the control group (↑61.38%, $p \leq 0.0001$) and in the group of psoriasis patients with normal salivation (↑30.47%, $p = 0.009$). The concentration of IL-10 (↓25.68%, $p = 0.002$; ↓47.30%, $p \leq 0.0001$, respectively) in the NWS of psoriasis patients with normal and decreased saliva secretion was considerably lower than in the control group. Moreover, the concentration of IL-10 (↓29.09%, $p = 0.03$) in NWS of patients with hyposalivation was significantly lower than in the group of psoriasis patients with normal saliva secretion (Figure 1).

3.1.2. SWS

TNF-α concentration (↑69.77%, $p \leq 0.0001$; ↑103.32%, $p \leq 0.0001$, respectively) and IL-2 (↑45.10%, $p \leq 0.0001$; ↑67.65%, $p \leq 0.0001$, respectively) in SWS of patients with psoriasis with normal and decreased saliva secretion was significantly higher than in the control group. The concentration of TNF-α (↑19.77%, $p = 0.0002$) and IL-2 (↑15.54%, $p = 0.03$) in SWS of patients with hyposalivation was considerably higher than in psoriasis patients with normal saliva secretion. INF-γ content in SWS of psoriasis patients with hyposalivation was significantly higher than in the control group (↑66.28%, $p \leq 0.0001$) and in the group of psoriasis patients with normal saliva secretion (↑31.19%, $p = 0.03$). The level of IL-10 (↓44.23%, $p \leq 0.0001$; ↓61.54%, $p \leq 0.0001$, respectively) in SWS in psoriasis patients with normal and decreased saliva secretion was significantly lower than in the control group, with IL-10 content (↓31.23%, $p \leq 0.0001$; ↓61.54%, $p \leq 0.0001$, respectively) in SWS in hyposalivation patients significantly lower than in psoriasis patients with normal saliva secretion (Figure 1).

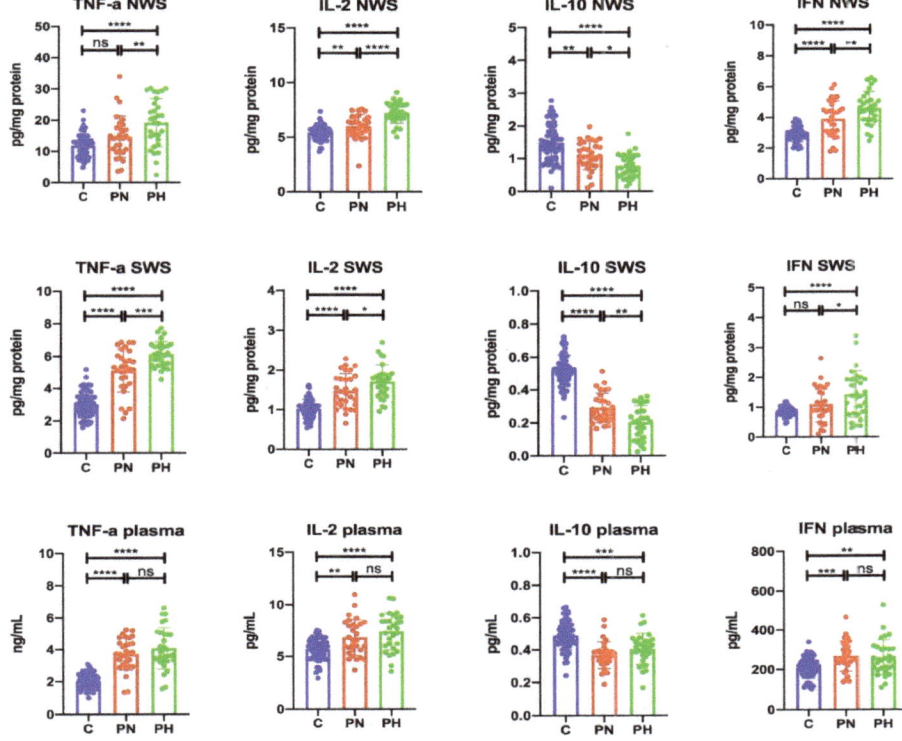

Figure 1. Cytokine levels in unstimulated and stimulated saliva as well as plasma of plaque psoriasis patients with normal salivation and hyposalivation. Abbreviations: C—the control; IL-2—interleukin 2; IL-10—interleukin-10; INF-γ—interferon-gamma; ns—not significant; NWS—non-stimulated whole saliva; PN—psoriasis patients with normal salivation; PH—psoriasis patients with hyposalivation; SWS—stimulated whole saliva; TNF-α—tumor necrosis factor-alpha. * $p < 0.05$, ** $p < 0.01$, *** $p < 0.001$, and **** $p < 0.0001$.

3.1.3. Plasma

TNF-α concentration in plasma of psoriasis patients with normal secretion (↑83.25%, $p \leq 0.0001$) and in plasma of psoriasis patients with hyposalivation (↑100.49%, $p \leq 0.0001$) was significantly higher than in the control group. Similarly, plasma concentration of IL-2 and INF-γ in psoriasis patients with normal secretion (↑19.68%, $p = 0.002$; ↑28.51%, $p = 0.0006$, respectively) and hyposalivation (↑29.70%, mboxemphp ≤ 0.0001; ↑25.29%, $p = 0.003$, respectively) were significantly higher vs. control. Plasma concentration of IL-10 in psoriasis patients with normal secretion (↓24.49%, $p \leq 0.0001$) and hyposalivation (↓18.37%, $p = 0.0001$) was significantly lower than in the control group (Figure 1).

3.2. Nitrosative Stress

3.2.1. NWS

The concentration of NO (↑14.31%, $p = 0.009$; ↑35.14%, $p \leq 0.0001$, respectively) and nitrotyrosine (↑12.41%, $p = 0.04$; ↑39.60%, $p \leq 0.0001$, respectively) in NWS of psoriasis patients with normal secretion and with hyposalivation was significantly higher than in the control group. Moreover, the levels of NO (↑18.23%, $p = 0.0006$) and nitrotyrosine (↑24.19%, $p \leq 0.0001$) in NWS of patients with hyposalivation was considerably higher than in psoriasis patients with normal salivary secretion.

The concentration of S-nitrosothiols and peroxynitrite in NWS of psoriasis patients with hyposalivation was significantly higher than in the control group (↑11.59%, $p = 0.04$; ↑30.70%, $p \leq 0.0001$, respectively) and the group of psoriasis patients with normal salivation (↑16.64%, $p = 0.01$; ↑17.63%, $p = 0.003$, respectively) (Figure 2).

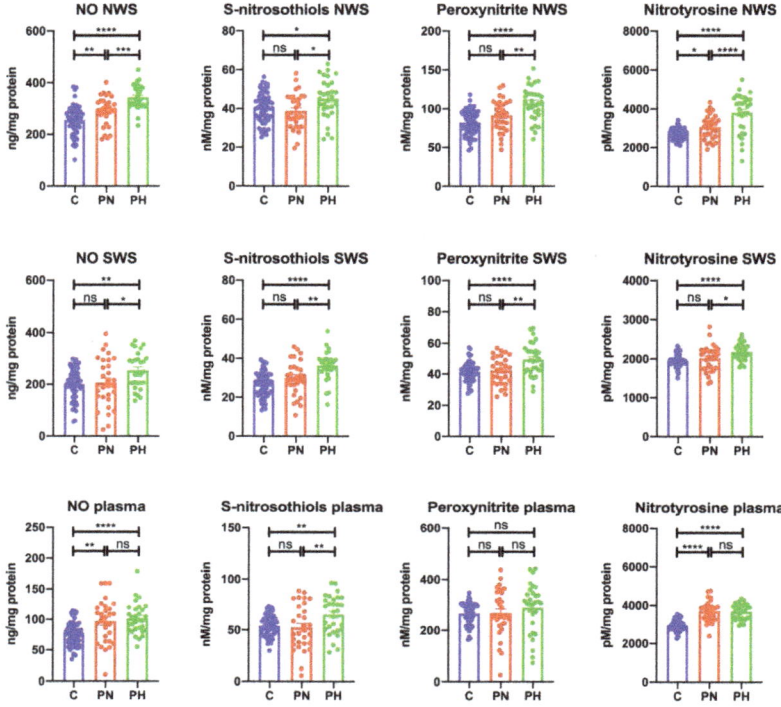

Figure 2. Nitrosative stress in non-stimulated and stimulated saliva as well as plasma of plaque psoriasis patients with normal salivation and hyposalivation. Abbreviations: C—the control; NO—nitric oxide; ns—not significant; NWS—non-stimulated whole saliva; PN—psoriasis patients with normal salivation; PH—psoriasis patients with hyposalivation; SWS—stimulated whole saliva. * $p < 0.05$, ** $p < 0.01$, *** $p < 0.001$, and **** $p < 0.0001$.

3.2.2. SWS

The concentration of NO, S-nitrosothiols, peroxynitrite, and nitrotyrosine in SWS of psoriasis patients with hyposalivation was significantly higher than in the control group (↑25.56%, $p = 0.006$; ↑35.93%, $p \leq 0.0001$; ↑11.47%, $p \leq 0.0001$; ↑11.80%, $p \leq 0.0001$, respectively), as well as compared to the group of psoriasis patients with normal salivation (↑22.71%, $p = 0.04$; ↑21.53%, $p = 0.002$; ↑17.26%, $p = 0.002$; ↑8.26%, $p = 0.02$, respectively) (Figure 2).

3.2.3. Plasma

The concentration of NO (↑27.19%, $p = 0.001$; ↑33.05%, $p \leq 0.0001$, respectively) and nitrotyrosine (↑25.04%, $p \leq 0.0001$; ↑24.34%, $p \leq 0.0001$, respectively) in plasma of psoriasis patients with normal and decreased saliva secretion was considerably higher than in the control group. Plasma concentration of S-nitrosothiols in psoriasis patients with hyposalivation was significantly higher than in the control group (↑20.41%, $p = 0.008$) and in psoriasis patients with normal saliva secretion (↑24.18%, $p = 0.008$). Plasma concentration of peroxynitrite did not differ between the study and control groups (Figure 2).

3.3. Salivary Gland Function

Unstimulated as well as stimulated saliva secretion was significantly lower in psoriasis patients with hyposalivation compared to the control group (↓57.58%, $p \leq 0.0001$; ↓41.03%, $p \leq 0.0001$, respectively). Similarly, unstimulated as well as stimulated saliva secretion was significantly lower in psoriasis patients with hyposalivation compared to the psoriatic patients with normal salivation (↓56.25%, $p \leq 0.0001$; ↓34.29%, $p = 0.0003$, respectively). The concentration of protein in NWS of psoriasis patients with hyposalivation was considerably lower than in the control group (↓24.90%, $p = 0.008$). Protein content in SWS of psoriasis patients with hyposalivation was significantly lower than in the controls (↓43.49%, $p \leq 0.0001$) and the group of patients with normal saliva secretion (↓13.60%, $p = 0.0008$). The activity of salivary amylase in NWS of psoriasis patients with hyposalivation and normal salivation was visibly lower than in the control group (↓30.00%, $p = 0.0003$; ↓25.00%, $p = 0.002$, respectively). Similarly, salivary amylase activity in SWS of psoriasis patients with hyposalivation and normal salivation was significantly lower than in the control group (↓42.86%, $p \leq 0.0001$; ↓25.00%, $p = 0.0006$, respectively). Moreover, amylase activity in SWS of patients with hyposalivation was considerably lower than in patients with normal salivation (↓23.81%, $p = 0.02$) (Figure 3).

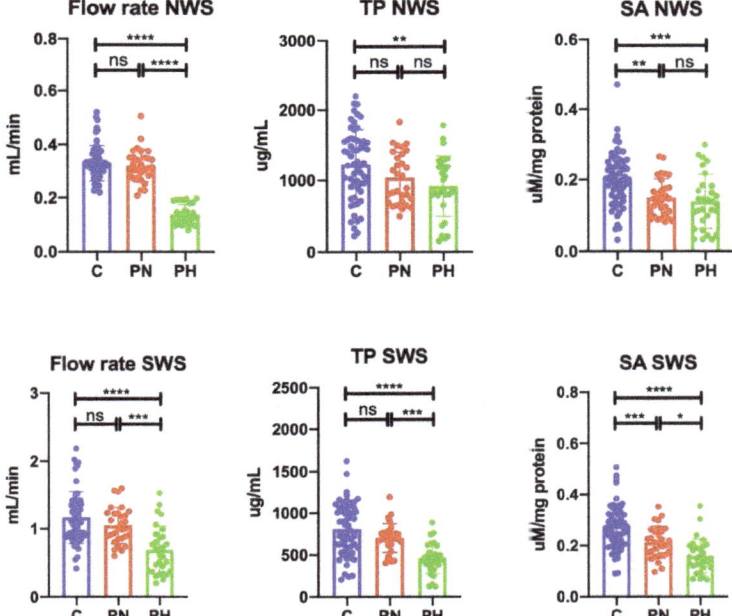

Figure 3. Salivary gland function in plaque psoriasis patients and control subjects. Abbreviations: C—the control; NWS—non-stimulated whole saliva; ns—not significant; PN—psoriasis patients with normal salivation; PH—psoriasis patients with hyposalivation; SA—salivary amylase; SWS—stimulated whole saliva; TP—total protein. * $p < 0.05$, ** $p < 0.01$, *** $p < 0.001$, and **** $p < 0.0001$.

3.4. ROC Analysis

The assessment of diagnostic usefulness of the analyzed biomarkers of inflammation and nitrosative stress is presented in Tables 2 and 3. Many of the assessed parameters clearly differentiated psoriatic patients with hyposalivation from patients with normal salivary flow. Particularly noteworthy is the assessment of NO, nitrotyrosine, and IL-2 levels in NWS, differentiating psoriatic patients with high sensitivity and specificity on the basis of the rate of saliva secretion (Figure 4).

Table 2. ROC analysis of the assessed cytokines and nitrosative stress biomarkers in the saliva of plaque psoriasis patients with normal salivation and hyposalivation.

Parameter	NWS							SWS				
	AUC	95% Confidence Interval	p-Value	Cut-Off	Sensitivity (%)	Specificity (%)	AUC	95% Confidence Interval	p-Value	Cut-Off	Sensitivity (%)	Specificity (%)	AUC
Cytokines												
TNF-α (pg/mg protein)	0.68	0.5417–0.8183	0.0166	>15.83	63.33	63.33	0.7311	0.6025–0.8597	0.0021	>5.717	66.67	66.67	0.5611
IL-2 (pg/mg protein)	0.8111	0.7024–0.9198	<0.0001	>6.789	73.33	73.33	0.6478	0.5071–0.7884	0.0493	>1.595	63.33	63.33	0.6122
IL-10 (pg/mg protein)	0.7089	0.5760–0.8418	0.0054	<0.9704	63.33	63.33	0.7267	0.5997–0.8536	0.0026	<0.2410	66.67	66.67	0.6556
INF-γ (pg/mg protein)	0.6622	0.5246–0.7999	0.0309	>4.358	60.00	60.00	0.6278	0.4848–0.7708	0.0891	>1.142	60.00	60.00	0.5378
Nitrosative Stress												
NO (ng/mg protein)	0.77	0.6507–0.8893	0.0003	>318.90	66.67	66.67	0.6464	0.5443–0.7885	0.0556	>224.00	60.71	60.00	0.5244
S-nitrosothiols (nM/mg protein)	0.6844	0.5479–0.8209	0.0141	>42.73	60.00	60.00	0.7211	0.5857–0.8565	0.0033	>34.60	70.00	70.00	0.6644
Peroxynitrite (nM/mg protein)	0.7056	0.5744–0.8367	0.0062	>101.50	63.33	63.33	0.69	0.5569–0.8231	0.0115	>45.31	60.00	60.00	0.5744
Nitrotyrosine (pM/mg protein)	0.7444	0.6120–0.8769	0.0011	>3398.00	70.00	70.00	0.6611	0.5223–0.8000	0.0321	>2139.00	60.00	60.00	0.5011

Abbreviations: AUC—area under the curve; C—the control; IL-2—interleukin 2; IL-10—interleukin 10; INF-γ—interferon-gamma; NO—nitric oxide; NWS—non-stimulated whole saliva; SWS—stimulated whole saliva; TNF-α—tumor necrosis factor-alpha.

Table 3. ROC analysis of the assessed cytokines and nitrosative stress biomarkers in the plasma of plaque psoriasis patients with normal salivation and hyposalivation.

Parameter	Plasma					
	AUC	95% Confidence Interval	p-Value	Cut-Off	Sensitivity (%)	Specificity (%)
Cytokines						
TNF-α (pg/mL)	0.5611	0.4135–0.7087	0.4161	>3.748	50.00	50.00
IL-2 (pg/mL)	0.6122	0.4685–0.7559	0.1354	>7.201	60.00	60.00
IL-10 (pg/mL)	0.6556	0.5127–0.7984	0.0385	>0.3863	63.33	63.33
INF-γ (pg/mL)	0.5378	0.3897–0.6858	0.6152	<251.20	50.00	50.00
Nitrosative Stress						
NO (ng/mg protein)	0.5244	0.3743–0.6746	0.745	>99.49	46.67	46.67
S-nitrosothiols (nM/mg protein)	0.6644	0.5261–0.8028	0.0287	>57.03	60.00	60.00
Peroxynitrite (nM/mg protein)	0.5744	0.4261–0.7228	0.3219	>302.90	60.00	60.00
Nitrotyrosine (pM/mg protein)	0.5011	0.3528–0.6494	0.9882	<3747.00	50.00	50.00

Abbreviations: AUC—area under the curve; C—the control; IL-2—interleukin 2; IL-10—interleukin 10; INF-γ—interferon-gamma; NO—nitric oxide; NWS—non-stimulated whole saliva; SWS—stimulated whole saliva; TNF-α—tumor necrosis factor-alpha.

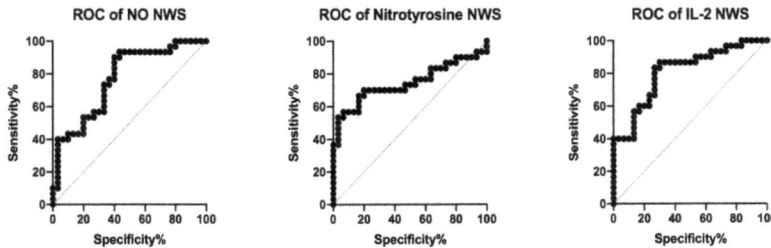

Figure 4. Receiver operating characteristic (ROC) analysis of nitric oxide, nitrotyrosine, and IL-2 in unstimulated saliva of plaque psoriasis patients with normal salivation and hyposalivation. IL-2—interleukin 2; NO—nitric oxide; NWS—non-stimulated whole saliva.

3.5. Correlations

The results of statistically significant correlations are presented in Table 4. We demonstrated a negative correlation between NO concentration and minute secretion of unstimulated saliva as well as between peroxynitrite and protein concentrations in stimulated saliva of patients with hyposalivation. Moreover, we observed a negative correlation between TNF-α level and non-stimulated salivation, as well as in IL-2 content and stimulated salivary flow in patients with hyposalivation. On the other hand, peroxynitrite concentration correlated negatively with α-amylase activity in both unstimulated and stimulated saliva of patients with normal salivation.

We noted a positive correlation between TNF-α and NO concentrations in unstimulated saliva of patients with hyposalivation, as well as between IL-2 and NO contents in unstimulated saliva of psoriasis patients with normal saliva secretion.

We showed a positive correlation between PASI and TNF-α, as well as PASI and IL-2 in unstimulated saliva of patients with hyposalivation. Moreover, we observed a positive correlation between nitrotyrosine concentration and duration of psoriasis in patients with normal as well as reduced salivary flow (both in unstimulated and stimulated saliva).

Table 4. Statistically significant correlations in patients with plaque psoriasis.

Pair of Variables	Group	r	p
NO NWS and NWS flow rate	PH	−0.68	0.001
Peroxynitrite SWS and total protein SWS	PH	−0.56	0.0015
TNF-α NWS and NWS flow rate	PH	−0.60	0.004
IL-2 SWS and SWS flow rate	PH	−0.54	0.002
Peroxynitrite NWS and amylase NWS	PN	−0.58	0.0008
Peroxynitrite SWS and amylase SWS	PN	−0.68	<0.0001
TNF-α NWS and NO NWS	PH	0.60	0.004
IL-2 NWS and NO NWS	PN	0.64	0.002
TNF-α NWS and PASI	PH	0.59	0.0006
IL-2 NWS and PASI	PH	0.63	0.0029
Nitrotyrosine NWS and disease duration	PN	0.53	0.003
Nitrotyrosine SWS and disease duration	PN	0.58	0.001
Nitrotyrosine NWS and disease duration	PH	0.61	0.004
Nitrotyrosine SWS and disease duration	PH	0.60	<0.0001

Abbreviations: IL-2—interleukin 2; NO—nitric oxide; NWS—non-stimulated whole saliva; PN—psoriasis patients with normal salivation; PH—psoriasis patients with hyposalivation; SWS—stimulated whole saliva; TNF-α—tumor necrosis factor-alpha.

4. Discussion

In the presented study, we evaluated the concentrations of TNF-α, IL-2, INF-γ, IL-10, and selected nitrosative stress parameters (NO, peroxynitrite, S-nitrosothiols, and nitrotyrosine) in NWS and SWS, as well as the plasma of psoriasis patients. The obtained results demonstrated the pathophysiology of salivary gland dysfunction in the course of plaque psoriasis. We were also seeking salivary psoriasis biomarkers that could be helpful in diagnosing the severity of psoriasis and its salivary complications.

The accepted values of normal unstimulated salivary flow are above 0.2 mL/min. Any unstimulated flow rate below 0.2 mL/min is considered salivary gland hypofunction and is referred to as hyposalivation [18]. Hyposalivation has a detrimental effect on numerous aspects of oral health, and thus on general well-being. It decreases the quality of life as it hinders speaking, tasting, chewing, and swallowing food [40]. Reduced saliva secretion is the cause of cracks and fissures in the oral mucosa, which is associated with chronic pain in the oral cavity and the resulting discomfort to the patient. Decreased salivation also contributes to boosted incidence of caries, periodontitis, and fungal infections of the oral cavity [40]. All these may lead to patient malnutrition, social isolation, and even depression, as well as generate high treatment costs. Therefore, it is very important to identify patients with salivation disorders and to prevent the development and effects of salivary gland dysfunction in the course of systemic diseases.

Our findings that plasma concentrations of TNF-α, IL-2, and INF-γ were significantly higher and for IL-10 were significantly lower than in the controls are consistent with the assumption that psoriasis is primarily driven by an aberrant immune response and results from an imbalance between Th1 and Th2 cells [2–4]. Significantly higher concentration of NO, especially nitrotyrosine, and a positive correlation between the latter and the disease duration in psoriatic patients' plasma compared to the controls confirm the contribution of nitrosative stress to the development of the disease [41]. Interestingly, apart from S-nitrosothiols, we did not observe significant differences between patients with hyposalivation and those with normal saliva secretion. On the other hand, patients from the hyposalivation group were characterized by longer duration of psoriasis and higher PASI index compared to those with normal flow of unstimulated saliva.

At this point, it is worth reminding that 90% of saliva is produced by three pairs of large salivary glands: submandibular, parotid, and sublingual. The remaining 10% of saliva is secreted by small salivary glands scattered under the oral cavity mucosa, and gingiva fluid. The submandibular glands are the major contributor to unstimulated salivary flow, and the parotid glands secrete stimulated saliva, that is, saliva secreted mainly in response to stimuli. The contribution of the sublingual glands to unstimulated and stimulated salivation is low [42]. Therefore, any deviation in the composition of unstimulated saliva reflects dysfunction of the submandibular glands, as well as of stimulated saliva, of the parotid glands. The exception here are patients with inflammatory changes in periodontal tissues, in whom changes in saliva composition reflect periodontal diseases. In our work, we excluded patients with periodontitis/gingivitis, and therefore any changes observed in saliva originated from the dysfunction of salivary glands.

Our results revealed significantly increased levels of the tested proinflammatory cytokines and a decrease in IL-10 concentration in unstimulated and stimulated saliva of psoriasis patients with normal salivation (except for TNF-α in NWS and INF-γ in SWS) and hyposalivation compared to the controls. An earlier report suggested that mRNA expression of Th1 and derived inflammatory cytokines IL-2, TNF-α, and INF-γ were also increased in the saliva of the patients with Sjögren's syndrome [43]. The salivary changes were accompanied by clusters of infiltrating cells present in salivary gland biopsy, where 80% were Th1 cells, and the remaining 20% consisted of stimulated B lymphocytes and plasma cells [43]. On the basis of the performed analyses, it was difficult to assess the nature of the developing inflammation in salivary glands of our patients. There were also no histological examinations of the salivary glands of psoriasis patients. By analogy to Sjögren's syndrome, the observed increases in TNF-α, IL-2, and INF-γ concentrations allow us to assume that salivary glands of patients with psoriasis are infested with autoreactive Th1 lymphocytes. Despite the deficiency of Th2 response (↓IL-10) supporting the humoral type response, we do not rule out the presence of stimulated B lymphocytes, as there has been no research to confirm or exclude the existence of the culprit autoantigens. However, increased concentration of the examined proinflammatory cytokines and decreased level of IL-10 in NWS and SWS of patients with hyposalivation compared to psoriasis patients with normal salivation indicates an increase in imbalance between Th1 and Th2 cells, and thus inflammation in salivary glands of patients with hyposalivation vs. those with normal salivary flow.

Human salivary glands contain different kinds of nitric oxide synthase (NOS) isoforms. Neuronal NOS (nNOS) was found in the salivary gland parenchyma, ducts, blood vessels, and nerve fibers around acini, mainly in the submandibular glands [44], and—in negligible amounts—in the parotid and sublingual glands [45]. Endothelial NOS (eNOS) was identified as localizing to the glandular vascular endothelium of the salivary ducts [45]. iNOS has been detected in the salivary ducts of normal tissue [45]. In physiological concentrations, NO does not damage the structures of salivary glands; it regulates oral blood flow and saliva secretion, and participates in non-specific protective mechanisms [23–25], which seems to take place in parotid glands of psoriasis patients without salivation disorders (no changes in the studied nitrosative stress parameters in SWS). We observed excessive amount of NO and peroxynitrite in unstimulated and stimulated saliva of patients with hyposalivation. A positive correlation between TNF-α and NO concentrations in NWS of patients with hyposalivation and between IL-2 and NO content in NWS of patients with normal salivation confirm the previous observations that proinflammatory cytokines lead to the expression of iNOS in salivary gland cells, resulting in increased production of NO and its derivatives [46]. We also noted a boost in nitrosative stress (NO, S-nitrosothiols, peroxynitrite) and, primarily, nitrosative damage to protein elements of the salivary glands (S-nitrosothiols and nitrotyrosine) in unstimulated and stimulated saliva of psoriasis patients with hyposalivation vs. those with normal saliva secretion.

Evidence has shown that much larger amounts of NO generated in response to inflammation are connected with the cytotoxic effect of NO due to its interaction with superoxide anions to form peroxynitrite and other free radicals. Research results have revealed that intense production of NO and peroxynitrite in salivary glands acts as a strong proapoptotic agent [46,47]. Moreover, it has been observed that NO, by auto-ADP (adenosyno-diphospate) ribosylation of glyceraldehyde 3-phosphate dehydrogenase, inhibits the production of ATP that is necessary to maintain anabolic processes in the cell [23]. It has been demonstrated that apoptosis of salivary gland structures disturbs their function, and ATP deficiency impairs mechanisms responsible for replacing damaged or lost cellular elements [46,48]. We noted a negative correlation between NO and NWS secretion, and between peroxynitrite and protein concentrations in SWS of hyposalivation patients. These results suggest that decreased salivary secretion and protein synthesis/selection could be caused by the proapoptotic effect of NO on the salivary gland cells. This hypothesis requires further confirmation in histological studies. On the other hand, it is known that TNF-α and IL-2 stimulate the production of metalloproteinases, which results in structural changes in the basement membrane of the salivary glands [49]. A negative correlation between TNF-α and NWS secretion, and IL-2 and SWS secretion in patients with hyposalivation may result from damage to acinar cell-basement membrane interaction resulting from overproduction of MMPs (metalloproteinases) followed by decreased number of secretory units (acini and ducts) [50,51]. This phenomenon has been recently demonstrated in the saliva of Sjögren's syndrome patients [52]. Remodeling of the extracellular matrix, alongside apoptosis, could be the reason for the observed drop in the synthesis/secretion of proteins and reduced salivary secretion in psoriasis patients with hyposalivation. It is noteworthy that salivary gland dysfunction occurs in patients with a longer duration and higher intensity of the disease.

The lack of significant differences in the secretion of NWS and SWS as well as proteins between patients with normal salivation (shorter disease duration, lower PASI) and the controls suggests that, at an early stage of the disease, the mechanisms of controlling saliva secretion and protein production/secretion counteract the damaging effects of psoriasis. Interestingly, already at this early stage we observed decreased amylase activity in SWS and UWS of patients with normal salivation, as well as intensification of this phenomenon in the saliva of patients with hyposalivation. These results may explain the negative correlation between peroxynitrite concentration and salivary amylase activity in NWS and SWS of patients with normal salivation. It has been demonstrated that peroxynitrite reacts readily with iron-sulfur cluster of several enzymes and is able to oxidize the sulfhydryl groups of proteins, leading to the formation of disulfides and resulting in their inactivation [53]. Naturally, it should be remembered that exposure to peroxynitrite entails tyrosine nitration of proteins [54]. This mechanism of amylase inactivation should be eliminated, as increased nitrotyrosine concentration was only observed in NWS and SWS of patients with hyposalivation, both compared to the controls and patients with normal saliva secretion.

Salivary glands are surrounded by a dense network of blood vessels that enable the exchange of components between the acinar cells and ducts, as well as blood. Thus, biomarkers present in the blood can permeate into the structures of salivary glands and hence into saliva. Therefore, saliva is more and more frequently considered a potential source of biological markers for systemic diseases. Many of the examined parameters clearly differentiated psoriatic patients with hyposalivation from psoriatic patients with normal saliva flow, and thus the levels of NO, nitrotyrosine, and IL-2 in NWS deserve special attention and should be further evaluated. Additionally, the observed positive correlation of PASI and TNF-α and IL-1β in UWS of patients with hyposalivation could provide a new non-invasive and simple method in the diagnosis of the intensity of the disease.

5. Conclusions

Increased levels of TNF-α, IL-2, and INF-γ, as well as decreased content of IL-10 in NWS and SWS of psoriasis patients compared to the controls indicated an imbalance between Th1 and Th2 cells in the salivary glands.

The severity of inflammation and nitrosative stress in the salivary glands of psoriatic patients depends on the disease duration.

At an early stage of the disease, the mechanisms controlling saliva secretion and protein production/secretion counteract the damaging effects of psoriasis. With the severity and duration of psoriasis, the secretory function of all salivary glands is lost, which is manifested as significant reduction of unstimulated and stimulated saliva secretion as well as protein concentration.

Dysfunction of salivary glands in the course of psoriasis may be attributed to inflammation and nitrosative stress.

Author Contributions: Conceptualization, A.Z., M.M.; data curation, A.S.-R., U.K., A.K., A.K.-R., J.K.; formal analysis, A.Z., M.M., A.S.-R.; funding acquisition, A.S.-R., A.Z.; investigation, A.S.-R., A.Z., M.M.; methodology, A.Z., M.M.; material collection: A.S.-R., U.K., A.K., A.K.-R.; supervision, A.Z., I.F., J.K.; validation, A.S.-R., A.Z., M.M.; visualization, M.M.; writing—original draft, A.S.-R., A.Z., M.M.; writing—review and editing, A.Z., M.M. All authors have read and agreed to the published version of the manuscript.

Funding: This work was supported by grants from the Medical University of Bialystok, Poland (grant numbers: SUB/1/DN/20/002/1209; SUB/1/DN/20/002/3330).

Conflicts of Interest: The authors declare no conflict of interest.

References

1. WHO. *Global Report on Psoriasis*; WHO Library Cataloguing-in-Publication Data; World Health Organization: Geneva, Switzerland, 2016; pp. 10–11.
2. Kupper, T.S. Immunologic Targets in Psoriasis. *N. Engl. J. Med.* **2003**, *349*, 1987–1990. [CrossRef] [PubMed]
3. Nickoloff, B.J. The immunologic and genetic basis of psoriasis. *Arch. Dermatol.* **1999**, *135*, 1104–1110. [CrossRef] [PubMed]
4. Liu, R.; Yang, Y.; Yan, X.; Zhang, K. Abnormalities in cytokine secretion from mesenchymal stem cells in psoriatic skin lesions. *Eur. J. Dermatol.* **2013**, *23*, 600–607. [CrossRef]
5. Asha, K.; Singal, A.; Sharma, S.B.; Arora, V.K.; Aggarwal, A. Dyslipidaemia & oxidative stress in patients of psoriasis: Emerging cardiovascular risk factors. *Indian J. Med. Res.* **2017**, *146*, 708–713. [PubMed]

6. Kadam, D.P.; Suryakar, A.N.; Ankush, R.D.; Kadam, C.Y.; Deshpande, K.H. Role of oxidative stress in various stages of psoriasis. *Indian J. Clin. Biochem.* **2010**, *25*, 388–392. [CrossRef]
7. Houshang, N.; Reza, K.; Sadeghi, M.; Ali, E.; Mansour, R.; Vaisi-Raygani, A. Antioxidant status in patients with psoriasis. *Cell Biochem. Funct.* **2014**, *32*, 268–273. [CrossRef]
8. Pujari, V.K.M. The Serum Levels of Malondialdehyde, Vitamin E and Erythrocyte Catalase Activity in Psoriasis Patients. *J. Clin. Diagn. Res.* **2014**, *8*, CC14–CC16. [CrossRef]
9. Yildirim, M.; Inaloz, H.S.; Baysal, V.; Delibas, N. The role of oxidants and antioxidants in psoriasis. *J. Eur. Acad. Dermatol. Venereol.* **2003**, *17*, 34–36. [CrossRef]
10. Barygina, V.V.; Becatti, M.; Soldi, G.; Prignano, F.; Lotti, T.; Nassi, P.; Wright, D.; Taddei, N.; Fiorillo, C. Altered redox status in the blood of psoriatic patients: Involvement of NADPH oxidase and role of anti-TNF-α therapy. *Redox Rep.* **2013**, *18*, 100–106. [CrossRef]
11. Ferretti, G.; Bacchetti, T.; Campanati, A.; Simonetti, O.; Liberati, G.; Offidani, A. Correlation between lipoprotein (a) and lipid peroxidation in psoriasis: Role of the enzyme paraoxonase-1. *Br. J. Dermatol.* **2012**, *166*, 204–207. [CrossRef]
12. Drewa, G.; Krzyzynska-Malinowska, E.; Wozniak, A.; Protas-Drozd, F.; Mila-Kierzenkowska, C.; Rozwodowska, M.; Kowaliszyn, B.; Czajkowski, R. Activity of superoxide dismutase and catalase and the level of lipid peroxidation products reactive with TBA in patients with psoriasis. *Med. Sci. Monit.* **2002**, *8*, BR338–BR343. [PubMed]
13. Lin, X.; Huang, T. Oxidative stress in psoriasis and potential therapeutic use of antioxidants. *Free Radic. Res.* **2016**, *50*, 585–595. [CrossRef] [PubMed]
14. Aparicio, V.A.; Nebot, E.; Porres, J.M.; Sánchez, C.; Aranda, P.; Garcia-del Moral, R.; Machado-Vílchez, M. High-protein diets and renal status in rats. *Nutr. Hosp.* **2013**, *28*, 232–237. [PubMed]
15. Skutnik-Radziszewska, A.; Maciejczyk, M.; Fejfer, K.; Krahel, J.; Flisiak, I.; Kołodziej, U.; Zalewska, A. Salivary Antioxidants and Oxidative Stress in Psoriatic Patients: Can Salivary Total Oxidant Status and Oxidative Status Index Be a Plaque Psoriasis Biomarker? *Oxidative Med. Cell. Longev.* **2020**. [CrossRef] [PubMed]
16. Sondermann, W.; Djeudeu Deudjui, D.A.; Körber, A.; Slomiany, U.; Brinker, T.J.; Erbel, R.; Moebus, S. Psoriasis, cardiovascular risk factors and metabolic disorders: Sex-specific findings of a population-based study. *J. Eur. Acad. Dermatol. Venereol.* **2019**. [CrossRef] [PubMed]
17. Ungprasert, P.; Raksasuk, S. Psoriasis and risk of incident chronic kidney disease and end-stage renal disease: A systematic review and meta-analysis. *Int. Urol. Nephrol.* **2018**, *50*, 1277–1283. [CrossRef]
18. Zalewska, A.; Knaś, M.; Gińdzieńska-Sieśkiewicz, E.; Waszkiewicz, N.; Klimiuk, A.; Litwin, K.; Sierakowski, S.; Waszkiel, D. Salivary antioxidants in patients with systemic sclerosis. *J. Oral Pathol. Med.* **2014**, *43*, 61–68. [CrossRef]
19. Desoutter, A.; Soudain-Pineau, M.; Munsch, F.; Mauprivez, C.; Dufour, T.; Coeuriot, J.L. Xerostomia and medication: A cross-sectional study in long-term geriatric wards. *J. Nutr. Health Aging* **2012**, *16*, 575–579. [CrossRef]
20. Zalewska, A.; Knaś, M.; Waszkiewicz, N.; Waszkiel, D.; Sierakowski, S.; Zwierz, K. Rheumatoid arthritis patients with xerostomia have reduced production of key salivary constituents. *Oral Surg. Oral Med. Oral Pathol. Oral Radiol.* **2013**, *115*, 483–490. [CrossRef]
21. Ganzetti, G.; Campanati, A.; Santarelli, A.; Pozzi, V.; Molinelli, E.; Minnetti, I.; Brisigotti, V.; Procaccini, M.; Emanuelli, M.; Offidani, A. Involvement of the oral cavity in psoriasis: Results of a clinical study. *Br. J. Dermatol.* **2015**, *172*, 282–285. [CrossRef]
22. Stichtenoth, D.O.; Frölich, J.C. Nitric oxide and inflammatory joint diseases. *Br. J. Rheumatol.* **1998**, *37*, 246–257. [CrossRef] [PubMed]
23. Brune, B.; Lapetina, E.G. Activation of a cytosolic ADP-ribosyltransferase by nitric oxide-generating agents. *J. Biol. Chem.* **1989**, *264*, 8455–8458. [PubMed]
24. Modin, A.; Weitzberg, E.; Hökfelt, T.; Lundberg, J.M. Nitric oxide synthase in the pig autonomic nervous system in relation to the influence of NG-nitro-L-arginine on sympathetic and parasympathetic vascular control In Vivo. *Neuroscience* **1994**, *62*, 189–203. [CrossRef]
25. Toda, N.; Ayajiki, K.; Okamura, T. Neurogenic and endothelial nitric oxide regulates blood circulation in lingual and other oral tissues. *J. Cardiovasc. Pharmacol.* **2012**, *60*, 100–108. [CrossRef] [PubMed]

26. Asa'ad, F.; Fiore, M.; Alfieri, A.; Pigatto, P.D.M.; Franchi, C.; Berti, E.; Maiorana, C.; Damiani, G. Saliva as a Future Field in Psoriasis Research. *Biomed Res. Int.* **2018**. [CrossRef]
27. Villanova, F.; Di Meglio, P.; Nestle, F.O. Biomarkers in psoriasis and psoriatic arthritis. *Ann. Rheum. Dis.* **2013**, *72*, 104–110. [CrossRef]
28. Klimiuk, A.; Maciejczyk, M.; Choromańska, M.; Fejfer, K.; Waszkiewicz, N.; Zalewska, A. Salivary Redox Biomarkers in Different Stages of Dementia Severity. *J. Clin. Med.* **2019**, *8*, 840. [CrossRef]
29. Brandtzaeg, P. Do salivary antibodies reliably reflect both mucosal and systemic immunity? *Proc. Ann. N. Y. Acad. Sci.* **2007**, *1098*, 288–311. [CrossRef]
30. Choromańska, M.; Klimiuk, A.; Kostecka-Sochoń, P.; Wilczyńska, K.; Kwiatkowski, M.; Okuniewska, N.; Waszkiewicz, N.; Zalewska, A.; Maciejczyk, M. Antioxidant defence, oxidative stress and oxidative damage in saliva, plasma and erythrocytes of dementia patients. Can salivary AGE be a marker of dementia? *Int. J. Mol. Sci.* **2017**, *18*, 2205. [CrossRef]
31. Maciejczyk, M.; Szulimowska, J.; Skutnik, A.; Taranta-Janusz, K.; Wasilewska, A.; Wiśniewska, N.; Zalewska, A. Salivary Biomarkers of Oxidative Stress in Children with Chronic Kidney Disease. *J. Clin. Med.* **2018**, *7*, 209. [CrossRef]
32. Maciejczyk, M.; Szulimowska, J.; Taranta-Janusz, K.; Werbel, K.; Wasilewska, A.; Zalewska, A. Salivary FRAP as a marker of chronic kidney disease progression in children. *Antioxidants* **2019**, *8*, 409. [CrossRef]
33. Maciejczyk, M.; Zalewska, A.; Ładny, J.R. Salivary Antioxidant Barrier, Redox Status, and Oxidative Damage to Proteins and Lipids in Healthy Children, Adults, and the Elderly. *Oxid. Med. Cell. Longev.* **2019**. [CrossRef]
34. Hefti, A.F. Periodontal probing. *Crit. Rev. Oral Biol. Med.* **1997**, *8*, 336–356. [CrossRef]
35. Grisham, M.B.; Johnson, G.G.; Lancaster, J.R. Quantitation of nitrate and nitrite in extracellular fluids. *Methods Enzymol.* **1996**, *268*, 237–246.
36. Wink, D.A.; Kim, S.; Coffin, D.; Cook, J.C.; Vodovotz, Y.; Chistodoulou, D.; Jourd'heuil, D.; Grisham, M.B. Detection of S-nitrosothiols by fluorometric and colorimetric methods. *Methods Enzymol.* **1999**, *301*, 201–211.
37. Borys, J.; Maciejczyk, M.; Antonowicz, B.; Sidun, J.; Świderska, M.; Zalewska, A. Free radical production, inflammation and apoptosis in patients treated with titanium mandibular fixations—An observational study. *Front. Immunol.* **2019**. [CrossRef] [PubMed]
38. Beckman, J.S.; Ischiropoulos, H.; Zhu, L.; van der Woerd, M.; Smith, C.; Chen, J.; Harrison, J.; Martin, J.C.; Tsai, M. Kinetics of superoxide dismutase- and iron-catalyzed nitration of phenolics by peroxynitrite. *Arch. Biochem. Biophys.* **1992**, *298*, 438–445. [CrossRef]
39. Maciejczyk, M.; Kossakowska, A.; Szulimowska, J.; Klimiuk, A.; Knaś, M.; Car, H.; Niklińska, W.; Ładny, J.R.; Chabowski, A.; Zalewska, A. Lysosomal Exoglycosidase Profile and Secretory Function in the Salivary Glands of Rats with Streptozotocin-Induced Diabetes. *J. Diabetes Res.* **2017**. [CrossRef]
40. Jankowska, A.K.; Waszkiel, D.; Kobus, A.; Zwierz, K. Saliva as a main component of oral cavity ecosystem. Part II. Defense mechanisms. *Wiad. Lek.* **2007**, *60*, 253–257.
41. Dilek, N.; Dilek, A.R.; Taskin, Y.; Erkinüresin, T.; Yalçin, Ö.; Saral, Y. Contribution of myeloperoxidase and inducible nitric oxide synthase to pathogenesis of psoriasis. *Postepy Dermatol. Alergol.* **2016**, *33*, 435–439. [CrossRef] [PubMed]
42. Dawes, C.; Pedersen, A.M.L.; Villa, A.; Ekström, J.; Proctor, G.B.; Vissink, A.; Aframian, D.; McGowan, R.; Aliko, A.; Narayana, N.; et al. The functions of human saliva: A review sponsored by the World Workshop on Oral Medicine VI. *Arch. Oral Biol.* **2015**, *60*, 863–874. [CrossRef] [PubMed]
43. Fox, R.I.; Kang, H.I.; Ando, D.; Abrams, J.; Pisa, E. Cytokine mRNA expression in salivary gland biopsies of Sjögren's syndrome. *J. Immunol.* **1994**, *152*, 5532–5539. [PubMed]
44. Looms, D.; Tritsaris, K.; Pedersen, A.M.; Nauntofte, B.; Dissing, S. Nitric oxide signalling in salivary glands. *J. Oral Pathol. Med.* **2002**, *31*, 569–584. [CrossRef] [PubMed]
45. Soinila, J.; Nuorva, K.; Soinila, S. Nitric oxide synthase in human salivary glands. *Histochem. Cell Biol.* **2006**. [CrossRef]
46. De La Cal, C.; Lomniczi, A.; Mohn, C.E.; De Laurentiis, A.; Casal, M.; Chiarenza, A.; Paz, D.; McCann, S.M.; Rettori, V.; Elverdín, J.C. Decrease in salivary secretion by radiation mediated by nitric oxide and prostaglandins. *Neuroimmunomodulation* **2006**, *13*, 19–27. [CrossRef]
47. Slomiany, B.L.; Slomiany, A. Nitric oxide interferes with salivary mucin synthesis: Involvement of ERK and p38 mitogen-activated protein kinase. *J. Physiol. Pharmacol.* **2002**, *53*, 325–336.

48. Zalewska, A.; Ziembicka, D.; Zendzian-Piotrowska, M.; MacIejczyk, M. The impact of high-fat diet on mitochondrial function, free radical production, and nitrosative stress in the salivary glands of wistar rats. *Oxid. Med. Cell. Longev.* **2019**. [CrossRef]
49. Azuma, M.; Aota, K.; Tamatani, T.; Motegi, K.; Yamashita, T.; Ashida, Y.; Hayashi, Y.; Sato, M. Suppression of tumor necrosis factor alpha-induced matrix metalloproteinase 9 production in human salivary gland acinar cells by cepharanthine occurs via down-regulation of nuclear factor kappaB: A possible therapeutic agent for preventing the destruction of the acinar structure in the salivary glands of Sjögren's syndrome patients. *Arthritis Rheum.* **2002**, *46*, 1585–1594.
50. Bozzato, A.; Burger, P.; Zenk, J.; Uter, W.; Iro, H. Salivary gland biometry in female patients with eating disorders. *Eur. Arch. Oto Rhino Laryngol.* **2008**, *265*, 1095–1102. [CrossRef]
51. Heo, M.S.; Lee, S.C.; Lee, S.S.; Choi, H.M.; Choi, S.C.; Park, T.W. Quantitative analysis of normal major salivary glands using computed tomography. *Oral Surg. Oral Med. Oral Pathol. Oral Radiol. Endod.* **2001**, *92*, 240–244. [CrossRef]
52. Hanemaaijer, R.; Visser, H.; Konttinen, Y.T.; Koolwijk, P.; Verheijen, J.H. A novel and simple immunocapture assay for determination of gelatinase-B (MMP-9) activities in biological fluids: Saliva from patients with Sjögren's syndrome contain increased latent and active gelatinase-B levels. *Matrix Biol.* **1998**, *17*, 657–665. [CrossRef]
53. Weiner, D.; Khankin, E.V.; Levy, Y.; Reznick, A.Z. Effects of cigarette smoke borne reactive nitrogen species on salivary alpha-amylase activity and protein modifications. *J. Physiol. Pharmacol.* **2009**, *60*, 127–132. [PubMed]
54. Gryka, D.; Pilch, W.B.; Czerwińska-Ledwig, O.M.; Piotrowska, A.M.; Klocek, E.; Bukova, A. The influence of Finnish sauna treatments on the concentrations of nitric oxide, 3-nitrotyrosine and selected markers of oxidative status in training and non-training men. *Int. J. Occup. Med. Environ. Health* **2020**. [CrossRef] [PubMed]

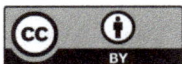

© 2020 by the authors. Licensee MDPI, Basel, Switzerland. This article is an open access article distributed under the terms and conditions of the Creative Commons Attribution (CC BY) license (http://creativecommons.org/licenses/by/4.0/).

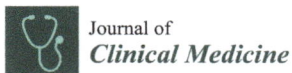

Article

Dysfunction of Salivary Glands, Disturbances in Salivary Antioxidants and Increased Oxidative Damage in Saliva of Overweight and Obese Adolescents

Anna Zalewska [1,*], Agnieszka Kossakowska [1], Katarzyna Taranta-Janusz [2], Sara Zięba [3], Katarzyna Fejfer [4], Małgorzata Salamonowicz [4], Paula Kostecka-Sochoń [4], Anna Wasilewska [2] and Mateusz Maciejczyk [5,*]

1. Experimental Dentistry Laboratory, Medical University of Bialystok, 15-222 Bialystok, Poland; a_kossak@op.pl
2. Department of Pediatrics and Nephrology, Medical University of Bialystok, 15-222 Bialystok, Poland; katarzyna.taranta@wp.pl (K.T.-J.); annwasil@interia.pl (A.W.)
3. Students Scientific Club "Biochemistry of Civilization Diseases" at the Department of Hygiene, Epidemiology and Ergonomics, Medical University of Bialystok, 15-222 Bialystok, Poland; sarap.zieba@gmail.com
4. Conservative Dentistry Department, Medical University of Bialystok, 15-222 Bialystok, Poland; katarzyna.fejfer@gmail.com (K.F.); wrobmalg@gmail.com (M.S.); p.kosta@wp.pl (P.K.-S.)
5. Department of Hygiene, Epidemiology and Ergonomics, Medical University of Bialystok, 15-222 Bialystok, Poland
* Correspondence: azalewska426@gmail.com (A.Z.); mat.maciejczyk@gmail.com (M.M.)

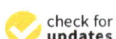

Received: 17 January 2020; Accepted: 14 February 2020; Published: 17 February 2020

Abstract: Obesity is inseparably connected with oxidative stress. This process may disturb the functioning of the oral cavity, although the effect of oxidative stress on salivary gland function and changes in the qualitative composition of saliva are still unknown. Our study is the first to evaluate salivary redox homeostasis in 40 overweight and obese adolescents and in the age- and gender-matched control group. We demonstrated strengthening of the antioxidant barrier (↑superoxide dismutase, ↑catalase, ↑peroxidase, ↑uric acid, ↑total antioxidant capacity (TAC)) with a simultaneous decrease in reduced glutathione concentration in saliva (non-stimulated/stimulated) in overweight and obese teenagers compared to the controls. The concentration of the products of oxidative damage to proteins (advanced glycation end products), lipids (malondialdehyde, 4-hydroxynonenal) and DNA (8-hydroxydeoxyguanosine) as well as total oxidative status were significantly higher in both non-stimulated and stimulated saliva as well as plasma of overweight and obese adolescents. Importantly, we observed more severe salivary and plasma redox alterations in obese adolescents compared to overweight individuals. In the study group, we also noted a drop in stimulated salivary secretion and a decrease in total protein content. Interestingly, dysfunction of parotid glands in overweight and obese teenagers intensified with the increase of BMI. We also showed that the measurement of salivary catalase and TAC could be used to assess the central antioxidant status of overweight and obese adolescents.

Keywords: oxidative stress; antioxidants; saliva; salivary biomarkers; obesity

1. Introduction

Overweight/obesity is a social problem worldwide, characterized by an increase in body weight that results in excessive accumulation of fat [1]. In recent years, we have observed a steady growth in the frequency of overweight and obesity, observed not only among adults, but also children and adolescents [2]. This results from various genetic, environmental and economic (easy access to cheap and highly calorific food) factors as well as evolutionary conditioning (sedentary lifestyle, low physical activity, low energy expenditure) [1,3]. According to the latest WHO report, nearly 41 million children under 5 years of age are overweight or obese [4]. Interestingly, studies have shown that about 40% of overweight children will continue to gain weight during the puberty period, and about 80% of these obese teenagers will remain obese as adults [5]. Although obesity rates are higher in developed countries, more overweight or obese children live in developing countries, and this trend also applies to European countries.

It has been shown that obesity is associated with an increase in oxidative stress (OS). OS is a condition characterized by disturbed balance between the amount of reactive oxygen species (ROS) produced by the body and activity/concentration of antioxidants responsible for neutralizing ROS [6]. ROS are chemically reactive molecules which, when unbalanced, lead to oxidative modifications of proteins, lipids, carbohydrates and nucleic acids, resulting in obesity-related complications.

It should be emphasized that obesity has been recognized as a major underlying factor in the pathogenesis of serious OS-related health problems, such as hyperlipidemia [7], insulin resistance [8], hypertension [9], type 2 diabetes [10], cardiovascular diseases [7] and certain types of cancer [11]. Overweight/obesity has been shown to adversely affect the condition of the oral cavity, including salivary gland function [12–14]. The pathogenesis of salivary gland lesions in the course of obesity is not fully understood, although the influence of OS is emphasized. It has been demonstrated that adult morbid obesity is associated with disorders of antioxidant systems [15,16] and oxidative damage to salivary proteins, lipids, and DNA [17], while bariatric treatment generally lowers the levels of salivary oxidative damage. However, it does not rescue antioxidant capacity of non-stimulated and stimulated saliva [16,17].

Recently, more and more attention has been paid to the use of saliva in laboratory medical diagnostics, particularly in connection with pediatric diseases, as the collection of saliva samples is non-invasive and thus acceptable to children. It has been shown that proteins and other substances are transported to saliva from blood via the passive process of diffusion, ultrafiltration and active transport. The concentrations of numerous substances in saliva can be correlated with their concentrations in blood plasma, allowing for the use of saliva as an alternative diagnostic material. Moreover, the use of oxidative stress biomarkers is proposed in diagnosing patients with obesity due to the observed changes in enzymatic and non-enzymatic antioxidant levels as well as accumulation of protein and lipid oxidation products in plasma and saliva of obese patients [16,17].

There have been numerous studies on OS in saliva and blood of overweight and obese adults [15–18], whereas no research has been conducted to evaluate salivary redox markers and their usefulness in diagnosing adolescents with excessive body weight. Therefore, the aim of our work is to evaluate antioxidant systems as well as oxidative modifications of proteins and lipids in non-stimulated and stimulated saliva of overweight and obese adolescents.

2. Materials and Methods

2.1. Patients

The study was approved by the Ethics Committee at the Medical University of Bialystok, Poland (permission number R-I-002/43/2018). After explaining the purpose and methodology of the study to patients and their parents, written informed content was obtained from each parent/legal guardian.

Our study included adolescents aged 11–18: overweight with BMI z-score $\leq +1 + 2 <$ SD ($n = 20$, 10 teenagers) and obese with BMI z-score $\geq +2$ SD ($n = 20$, 10 teenagers).

The control group consisted of adolescents ($n = 40$, 20 teenagers) with normal body weight (BMI z-score $< -1 + 1 <$, matched by age and gender to the study group.

The adolescents included in the study group were recruited in the Department of Pediatrics and Nephrology of the Medical University of Bialystok, during routine follow-up visits, after performing a dental and biochemical blood test and meeting the conditions for inclusion/exclusion to the study.

The adolescents included in the control group were recruited during dental follow-up visits in the Children's Outpatient Dentistry Clinic (Specialist Dental Centre of the Medical University of Bialystok), initially based on BMI index and a health survey. Then, after obtaining the written consent of participants and their legal guardians, biochemical blood tests were performed. If the participants met the conditions for inclusion/exclusion in the study, they were finally included in the control group.

Patients from the study and control group were qualified by the same experienced pediatrician (K.T.J.) as well as a pediatric dentist (A.Z.). The control group consisted of patients of the Children's Outpatient Dentistry Clinic because, in the Pediatrics and Nephrology Clinic, there were only a few healthy controls that met the inclusion criteria for the study.

Clinical data of the subjects are presented in Table 1.

Table 1. Clinical characteristics of patients and healthy controls.

	C n = 40	OWT n = 20	OB n = 20
Age (years)	16 ± 2.0	16 ± 1.9	15.8 ± 2.2
Sex (male/female) n	20/20	10/10	10/10
Weight (kg)	55 ± 3.1	65 ± 10 *	90 ± 21 *
Height (cm)	167 ± 4.5	163 ± 12	162 ± 14
BMI (kg/m^2)	20 ± 1.5	28 ± 1.5 *	34 ± 2.7 *
cc BMI	50 ± 2.5	97 ± 1.2	99 ± 0.83
SDS BMI	0.5 ± 0.2	2.5 ± 0.28	3.9 ± 0.81
Systolic BP (mmHg)	109 ± 1.0	110 ± 1.2	111 ± 1.0
Diastolic BP (mmHg)	58 ± 4.2	73 ± 10	76 ± 9.8
WBC (thousand/µL)	5.8 ± 1.3	6.7 ± 2.2	6.7 ± 1.1
Hgb (g/dL)	13.9 ± 1.1	14 ± 1.2	14 ± 1.0
Hct (%)	42.0 ± 2.3	41 ± 3.3	42 ± 3.2
PLT (thousand/µL)	278 ± 46	294 ± 71	263 ± 48
sCre (mg/dL)	0.63 ± 0.1	0.64 ± 0.19	0.79 ± 0.56
Urea (mg/dL)	15.4 ± 3.6	24 ± 9.7 *	27 ± 13 *
HDL (mg/dL)	47 ± 2.2	52 ± 1.4	43 ± 8.1
LDL (mg/dL)	70 ± 5.2	87 ± 24	106 ± 21 *
Total cholesterol (mg/dL)	120 ± 9	132 ± 30	161 ± 39 *
TG (mg/dL)	68 ± 8	102 ± 75 *	139 ± 75 *
Glucose (mg/dL)	86 ± 5.3	86 ± 9.9	91 ± 5.4
eGFR (mL/min/1.73 m^2)	132 ± 10	120 ± 42	122 ± 43
IL-6 (pg/mL)	1.7 ± 0.71	2.3 ± 0.74	3 ± 1.13

Body weight, height and head and chest circumferences were measured by standard methods. BMI was calculated as weight (kg) divided by the square of height (m^2). BMI z-scores that reflect the standard deviation score (SD) for age- and gender-appropriate BMI distribution, were calculated according to the LMS method [19], using reference values from the WHO study [20]. Based on the international norms from the World Health Organization for age- (with an accuracy of 1 month) and gender-specific BMI, BMI cut-offs for children over 5 years of age were the following: overweight–BMI z-score ≤ + 1 + 2 < SD; obesity–BMI z-score ≥ + 2 SD [21].

The inclusion criteria were: adolescents of both sexes (in the case of girls, those who had had menarche) with full permanent dentition. On the day of material collection, the teenage girls were in the first phase of their menstrual cycle.

Patients with deciduous and mixed dentition, with gingivitis (gingival index, GI > 0.5) and pathological changes in the oral cavity mucosa were excluded from the study. Negative general medical history was a necessary factor to qualify for the experiment. The questionnaire completed by the patients included: infectious, autoimmune and metabolic diseases (type 2 diabetes) as well as hypertension, insulin resistance and diseases of respiratory, cardiovascular, digestive, genitourinary and coagulation systems. The exclusion criteria also covered inappropriate behavior and/or refusal to cooperate with the examiner. At least 3 months before the study, patients and the healthy controls had not taken any oral non-steroidal anti-inflammatory drugs, glucocorticosteroids, vitamins, other supplements, or antibiotics. The participants were non-smokers and did not drink alcohol more frequently than once a month.

2.2. Blood Collection

Blood was collected on an empty stomach, during routine examinations in the case of adolescents from the control group, and for the study groups: during admission to the Pediatric and Nephrology Clinic of the Medical University of Bialystok. Blood was collected in the amount of 10 mL using an S-Monovette® EDTA K3 tube (Sarstedt, Nümbrecht, Germany). After collection, the blood was centrifuged (3000 g, 10 min, 4 °C). No hemolysis was observed in any of the obtained plasma samples. Blood cell mass was rinsed 3 times with 0.9% NaCl, and then underwent osmotic lysis using 50 mM cold phosphate buffer (pH 7.4) 1:9 (v/v) [17]. To prevent sample oxidation, 0.5 M BHT (Sigma-Aldrich, Saint Louis, MO, USA; 10 µl/ml blood) was added to the plasma and red blood cell lysate [17]. Plasma and blood lysate were frozen (−82 °C). The samples were stored deep-frozen for no longer than 6 months.

2.3. Saliva Collection

Non-stimulated and stimulated saliva was collected by the spitting method between 7 and 8 a.m., one day after admission to the Pediatrics and Nephrology Clinic of the UMB or during a routine dental check-up. The time since the last meal, tooth-brushing and taking medications was at least 10 h. Samples were collected in a separate room to ensure comfort for the subjects. After rinsing the mouth with water, participants spat out non-stimulated saliva accumulated at the bottom of the oral cavity for 15 min. Stimulated saliva was collected after a 5-min break. Stimulation was performed by dropping 20 µl of 2% citric acid on the tongue every 20 s for 5 min. Both types of saliva were collected in test tubes placed on ice. To prevent sample oxidation, 0.5 M BHT (Sigma-Aldrich, Saint Louis, MO, USA; 10 µl/ml blood) was added to the saliva. After collecting the samples, the volume of saliva was measured in a calibrated pipette with accuracy of 100 µL and saliva flow rate was estimated. Saliva samples were centrifuged (3000 g, 20 min, 4 °C, MPW 351, MPW Med. Instruments, Warsaw, Poland) and then frozen (−82 °C). Frozen samples were stored for no longer than 6 months.

In each of the obtained saliva samples, the concentration of transferrin was determined by the ELISA test to identify samples contaminated with blood. Transferrin was not detected in any of the saliva samples (data not shown).

2.4. Dental Examination

Immediately after saliva collection, dental examination was performed by the selected dentists (K. F., M. S., P. K.-S.) in artificial light, using a mirror, an explorer and a periodontal probe (WHO, 621) in accordance with the WHO criteria. The dental examination included the evaluation of DMFT (decayed, missing, filled teeth) and GI (gingival index). The interrater reliability for DMFT was $r = 0.92$, and for GI was $r = 0.94$.

2.5. Biochemical Determination

The performed assays included: antioxidant enzymes (salivary peroxidase (Px), EC 1.11.1.7, catalase (CAT), EC 1.11.1.6 and superoxide dismutase (SOD), EC 1.15.1.1), non-enzymatic antioxidants (reduced glutathione (GSH), uric acid (UA) and albumin), redox status (total oxidant status (TOS), total antioxidant capacity (TAC) and oxidative stress index (OSI)), advanced glycation end products (AGE), malondialdehyde (MDA), 4-NHE-protein adduct (4-HNE) and 8-hydroxy-D-guanosine (8-OHdG). All results were standardized to mg of total protein. The total protein content was determined using the bicinchoninic acid (BCA) method and bovine serum albumin (BSA) as a standard (Thermo Scientific PIERCE BCA Protein Assay (Rockford, IL, USA).

In the saliva samples, we analyzed all redox biomarkers. In erythrocytes, antioxidant enzymes were assayed, while in the blood plasma we evaluated non-enzymatic antioxidants, redox status and oxidative damage products as well as interleukin-6 (IL-6) concentration. All assays were performed in duplicate samples (TOS in triplicate samples), and the absorbance/fluorescence of the samples was measured with an Infinite M200 PRO Multimode Microplate Reader (Tecan).

2.6. Antioxidant Enzymes

The activity of salivary peroxidase (Px, E.C. 1.11.1.7) was determined colorimetrically according to Mansson-Rahemtulla et al. [22] based on the reduction of 5,5′-dithiobis-(2-nitrobenzoic acid) (DTNB) to thionitrobenzoic acid, which then reacted with thiocyanate anions (SCN^-) formed as a result of potassium thiocyanate (KSCN) oxidation by Px. The absorbance was measured at a 412 nm wavelength. The activity of catalase (CAT, E.C. 1.11.1.6) was determined by the colorimetric method described by Aebi [23], based on the measurement of the hydrogen peroxide (H_2O_2) decomposition rate in phosphate buffer at pH 7.0. The absorbance was measured at 240 nm wavelength. One unit of CAT activity was defined as the amount of the enzyme that decomposes 1 mM H_2O_2 for 1 min. The activity of superoxide dismutase-1 (SOD, E.C. 1.15.1.1) was determined colorimetrically according to Misra and Fridovich [24] based on the measurement of cytoplasmic activity of the SOD subunit in the reaction of inhibiting the oxidation of epinephrine to adrenochrome at a 320 nm wavelength. It was assumed that one unit of SOD activity inhibits epinephrine oxidation in 50%.

2.7. Non-Enzymatic Antioxidants

The concentration of reduced glutathione (GSH) was determined colorimetrically based on DTNB reduction to 2-nitro-5-mercaptobenzoic acid under the influence of GSH contained in the assayed samples [25]. Absorbance changes were measured at 412 nm wavelength. Uric acid (UA) concentration was determined by the colorimetric method using a set of ready-made reagents (QuantiChrom TM Uric Acid Assay Kit DIUA-250, BioAssay System Harward, CA, USA). The method is based on the reaction of 2,4,6-tripyridyl-s-triazine with iron (3+) ions in the presence of UA contained in the samples. Changes in the absorbance of the resulting complex were measured at a 590 nm wavelength.

2.8. Redox Status

Total antioxidant capacity (TAC) was determined colorimetrically as described by Erel [26], based on the measurement of the ability to neutralize the radical cation $ABTS^{·+}$ [2,2-azino-bis-(3-ethylbenzothiazoline-6-sulfonate)] under the influence of antioxidants contained in the tested samples. Changes in the absorbance of $ABTS^{·+}$ solution were measured at a 660 nm wavelength. Total oxidant status (TOS) was determined using the colorimetric method described by Erel [27], based on the oxidation of iron (2+) ions to iron (3+) ions in the presence of oxidants contained in the sample, followed by the detection of Fe^{3+} ions by xylene orange. TOS concentration was calculated from the standard curve for hydrogen peroxide and presented in nM H_2O_2 equivalent/mg total protein. TOS determination was performed in triplicate samples. The oxidative stress index (OSI) was presented as the quotient of TOS to TAC and expressed in % [28,29].

2.9. Products of Oxidative Damage to Proteins and Lipids

The content of protein advanced glycation end products (AGE) was determined fluorimetrically by the method described by Kalousová et al. [30] based on the measurement of fluorescence of furyl-furanyl-imidazole (FFI), carboxymethyl lysine (CML), pyraline and pentosidine at the excitation wavelength 350 nm and emission wavelength 440 nm. To determine the AGE content, the samples were diluted in PBS buffer (0.02 M, pH 7.0) in a volume ratio of 1:5, and mixed thoroughly [31]. AGE content was determined in duplicate samples and expressed in fluorescence arbitrary units AFU/mg total protein. The concentration of malondialdehyde (MDA) was determined colorimetrically using thiobarbituric acid (TBA) [32]. The MDA reaction with TBA produces a colored adduct with the maximum absorption at 535 nm wavelength. The concentrations of 4-HNE and 8-OHdG were assessed by ELISA with commercial sets (Cell Biolabs, Inc. San Diego, CA, USA; USCN Life Science, Wuhan, China, respectively), following the manufacturer's instructions included in the package.

2.10. Statistical Analysis

Statistical analysis of the results was performed using GraphPad Prism 8 and Microsoft Excel 16.16.12 for MacOS. The D'Agostino–Pearson test and Shapiro–Wilk test were used to assess the distribution of the results. Individual groups were compared using the analysis of variance (ANOVA) followed by Tukey's honest significant difference test (Tukey's HSD test). The multiplicity adjusted p value was also calculated. Correlations between redox biomarkers were assessed based on the Pearson correlation coefficient. The results were presented as mean and standard deviation (SD) using tables or graphs. Diagnostic usefulness of the redox biomarkers was evaluated by means of receiver operating characteristic (ROC) analysis. Statistical significance was assumed at $p \leq 0.05$.

The number of subjects was determined based on our previous experiment, assuming that the power of the test would equal 0.9.

3. Results

3.1. General Characteristics

Stimulated secretion was significantly lower in the group of overweight and obese adolescents compared to the controls (↓40%, $p < 0.0001$; ↓51%, $p < 0.0001$, respectively). Teenagers with obesity secreted considerably less saliva after stimulation than their overweight peers (18%, $p = 0.004$). The secretion of non-stimulated saliva did not differ significantly between the study groups as well as in comparison with the control group (Table 2).

Table 2. Salivary flow rate, total protein and stomatological findings.

	C n = 40	O n = 20	OB n = 20
NWS (mL/min)	0.42 ± 0.05	0.39 ± 0.11	0.41 ± 0.11
SWS (mL/min)	1.5 ± 0.1	0.9 ± 0.2 *	0.74 ± 0.18 *#
TP NWS (μg/mL)	1291 ± 227	1167 ± 299	1139 ± 245
TP SWS (μg/mL)	986 ± 327	658 ± 208 *	598 ± 197 *
DMFT	6 ± 2	8 ± 3	8 ± 2
GI	0.1 ± 0.1	0.1 ± 0.15	0.1 ± 0.12

NWS- non-stimulated salivary flow rate, SWS- stimulated salivary flow rate, TP- total protein, C- control, OWT- overweight, OB- obese, DMFT= decay, missing, filling teeth, PBI- papilla bleeding index, GI- gingival index, * $p < 0.05$ vs. C; # $p < 0.05$ vs. OWT.

Total protein concentration in stimulated saliva of overweight and obese adolescents was significantly lower than in the control group (↓33%, $p = 0.0001$; 40%, $p < 0.0001$, respectively). Protein concentration in non-stimulated saliva did not differ significantly between the study groups and compared to the control group (Table 2).

Scatter plots for BMI and NWS/SWS flow rate are presented in Figure 1.

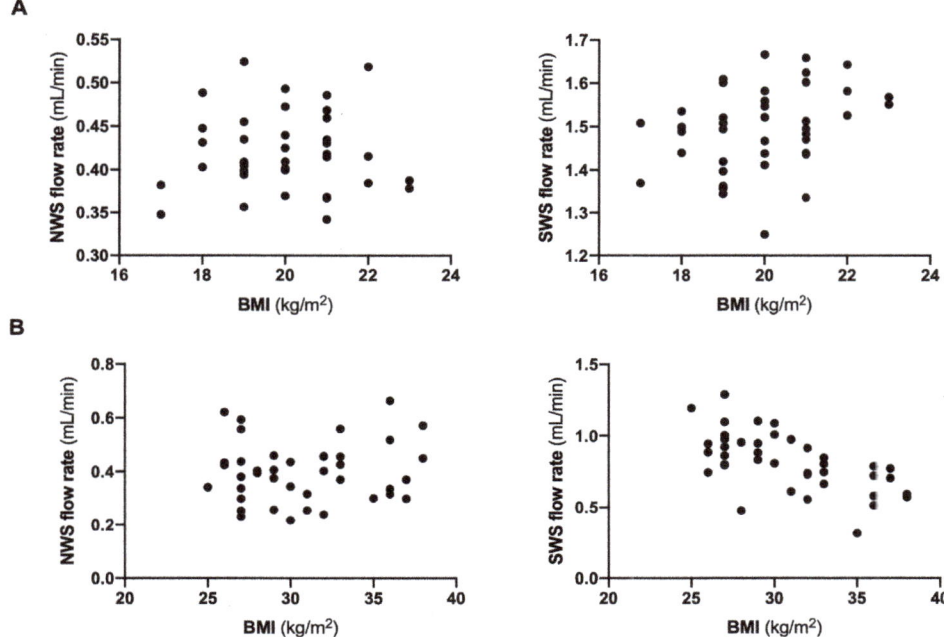

Figure 1. Scatter plots for BMI and non-stimulated and stimulated salivary flow rate in healthy children (**A**) as well as overweight and obese adolescents (**B**). BMI- body mass index; NWS- non-stimulated whole saliva; SWS- stimulated whole saliva.

There were no significant differences in the dental indexes DMFT and GI between the controls and the groups of overweight and obese adolescents (Table 2).

3.2. Enzymatic Antioxidants

The activity of SOD in non-stimulated and stimulated saliva of overweight adolescents was significantly higher than in the control group of adolescents with normal weight (↑60%, $p < 0.001$; ↑48%, $p = 0.002$, respectively). Similar significant differences were observed in the group of obese adolescents, in whom SOD activity in non-stimulated and stimulated saliva was significantly higher than in the control group (↑125%, $p < 0.001$; ↑78%, $p < 0.001$, respectively). There were no differences in salivary SOD activity between overweight and obese subjects. SOD activity in erythrocytes of both overweight (↓59%, $p < 0.001$) and obese (↓58%, $p < 0.001$) adolescents was considerably lower than in erythrocytes of teenagers with normal body weight, and did not differ between the study groups.

The activity of CAT in non-stimulated saliva of obese adolescents was significantly higher compared to the controls (↑75%, $p < 0.001$) and overweight adolescents (↑75%, $p < 0.001$).

The activity of CAT in stimulated saliva of overweight (↑62%, $p < 0.001$) and obese (↑90%, $p < 0.001$) adolescents was significantly higher than in the control group. CAT activity in erythrocytes of obese teenagers was considerably lower than in the control group (↓49%, $p < 0.001$) and in overweight adolescents (↓38%, $p = 0.02$).

The activity of Px in non-stimulated saliva did not differ between the study groups and the controls. Px activity in stimulated saliva and erythrocytes of overweight (↑78%, $p < 0.001$; ↑153%, $p < 0.001$, respectively) and obese (↑57%, $p < 0.001$; ↑153%, $p < 0.001$, respectively) adolescents was significantly higher than in saliva and erythrocytes of the control group (Figure 2).

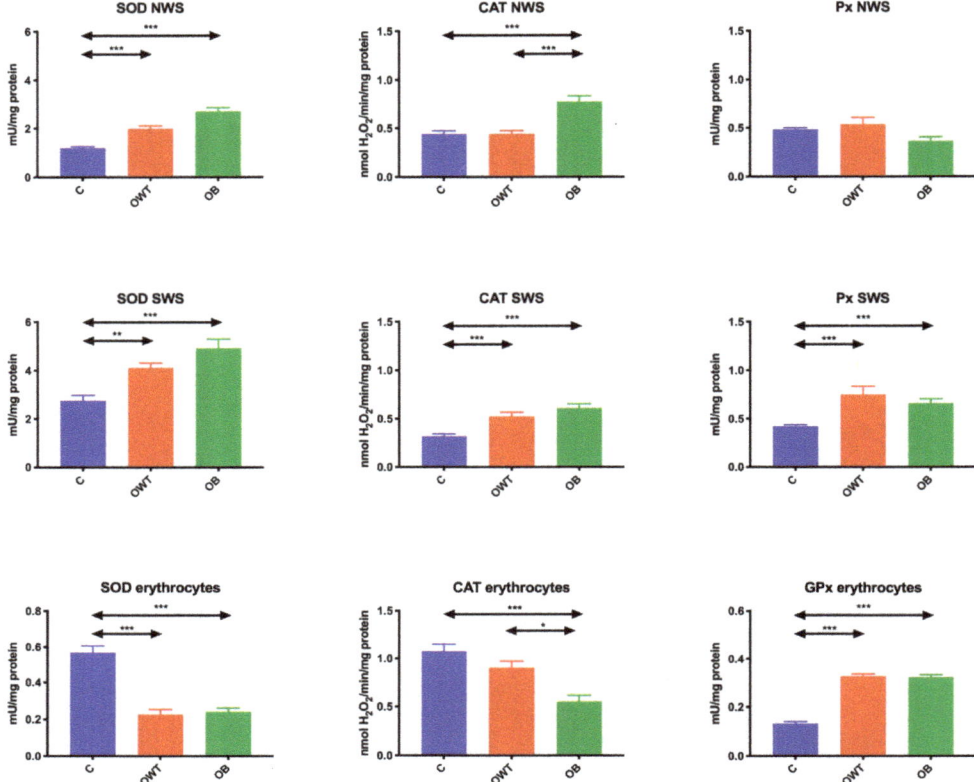

Figure 2. Enzymatic antioxidants in overweight and obese adolescents as well as healthy controls. C- control, CAT- catalase, NWS- non-stimulated whole saliva, OB- obese, OWT- overweight, Px- salivary peroxidase, SOD- superoxide dismutase, SWS- stimulated whole saliva. Differences statistically significant at: * $p < 0.05$, ** $p < 0.005$, *** $p < 0.0005$.

3.3. Non-Enzymatic Antioxidants

The concentration of GSH in non-stimulated and stimulated saliva of overweight (↓47%, $p < 0.001$; ↓26%, $p = 0.005$, respectively) and obese (↓65%, $p < 0.001$; ↓54%, $p < 0.001$, respectively) adolescents was significantly lower than in the control group. However, the GSH concentration in overweight adolescents was significantly higher only in stimulated saliva compared to obese subjects (↑38%, $p < 0.001$). Plasma GSH concentration in obese adolescents was significantly lower than in the control group (↓29%, $p < 0.006$).

The concentration of UA in non-stimulated saliva of obese adolescents was significantly higher than in the controls (↑37%, $p < 0.001$). UA concentration in stimulated saliva of overweight and obese adolescents was considerably higher than in the control group (↑157%, $p < 0.001$; ↑198%, $p < 0.001$, respectively). Plasma UA concentration in overweight and obese adolescents was significantly elevated compared to their peers with normal body weight (↑43%, $p < 0.001$; ↑45%, $p < 0.001$, respectively) (Figure 3).

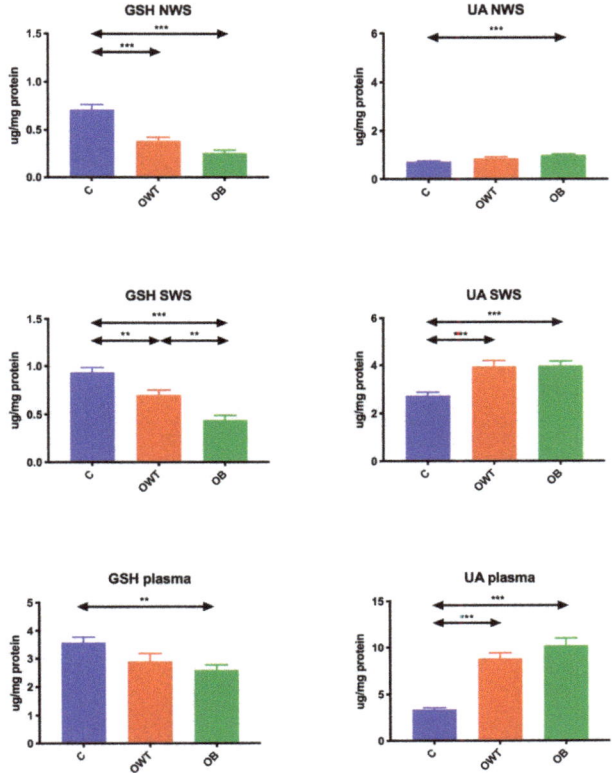

Figure 3. Non-enzymatic antioxidants in overweight and obese adolescents as well as healthy controls. C- control, GSH- reduced glutathione, NWS- non-stimulated whole saliva, OB- obese, OWT- overweight, SWS- stimulated whole saliva, UA- uric acid. Differences statistically significant at: ** $p < 0.005$, *** $p < 0.0005$.

3.4. Redox Status

In overweight and obese adolescents, TAC in non-stimulated (↑110%, $p < 0.001$; ↑122%, $p < 0.001$, respectively) and stimulated (↑62%, $p < 0.001$; ↑56%, $p < 0.001$, respectively) saliva as well as plasma (↑61%, $p < 0.001$; ↑75%, $p < 0.001$, respectively) was considerably higher than in the control group.

TOS in non-stimulated (↑113%, $p < 0.001$; ↑288%, $p < 0.001$, respectively) and stimulated (↑115%, $p < 0.001$; ↑170%, $p < 0.001$, respectively) saliva as well as plasma (↑103%, $p < 0.001$; ↑97%, $p \leq 0.001$, respectively) of overweight and obese adolescents was significantly raised compared to the control group. TOS in non-stimulated (↑129%, $p < 0.001$) and stimulated (↑25%, $p = 0.001$) saliva of obese teenagers was considerably higher than in their overweight peers.

OSI in non-stimulated and stimulated saliva as well as plasma in obese adolescents was significantly higher than in the controls (↑153%, $p < 0.001$; ↑105%, $p = 0.001$; ↑48%, $p = 0.01$, respectively) (Figure 4).

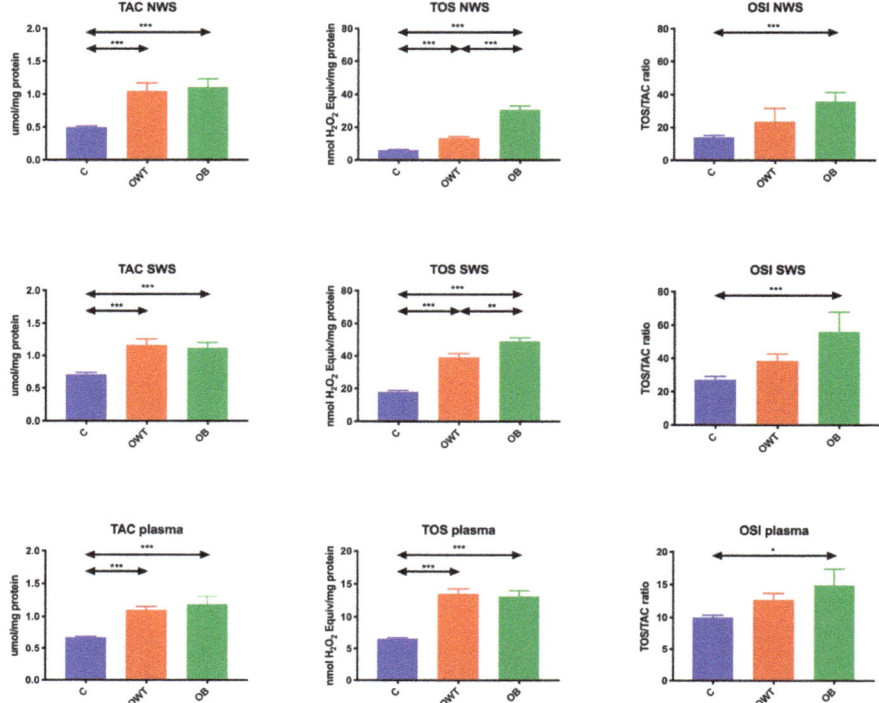

Figure 4. Redox status in overweight and obese adolescents as well as healthy controls. C- control, NWS- non-stimulated whole saliva, OB- obese, OSI- oxidative stress index, OWT- overweight, SWS- stimulated whole saliva, TAC- total antioxidant capacity, TOS- total oxidative status. Differences statistically significant at: * $p < 0.05$, ** $p < 0.005$, *** $p < 0.0005$.

3.5. Oxidation Products

AGEs in non-stimulated and stimulated saliva as well as plasma of both overweight (↑281%, $p < 0.001$; ↑209%, $p < 0.001$; ↑203%, $p < 0.001$, respectively) and obese (↑347%, $p < 0.001$; ↑423%, $p < 0.001$; ↑244%, $p < 0.001$, respectively) adolescents were significantly higher compared to the saliva of the control group. Only AGEs in stimulated saliva of obese adolescents were considerably higher than in overweight adolescents (↑69%, $p < 0.001$).

MDA in non-stimulated and stimulated saliva as well as plasma in both overweight (↑43%, $p < 0.001$; ↑63%, $p = 0.001$; ↑41%, $p < 0.001$, respectively) and obese (↑43%, $p < 0.001$; ↑79%, $p < 0.001$; ↑55%, $p < 0.001$, respectively) teenagers were significantly higher than in saliva of control group adolescents.

The concentration of 4-HNE was notably higher in non-simulated and stimulated saliva as well as plasma of overweight (33% $p = 0.01$; 50% $p < 0.001$; 41% $p = 0.003$) and obese adolescents (84% $p < 0.001$; 95% $p < 0.001$; 104% $p < 0.001$) compared to the control group. The concentration of 4-HNE in non-simulated and stimulated saliva as well as plasma of obese adolescents was considerably higher than in overweight adolescents (37% $p < 0.001$; 50% $p < 0.001$; 43% $p < 0.001$). Similarly, the concentration of 8-OHdG in non-simulated and stimulated saliva as well as plasma of both overweight (53% $p < 0.001$; 25% $p = 0.04$; 62% $p < 0.001$) and obese adolescents (121% $p < 0.001$; 73% $p < 0.001$; 118% $p < 0.001$) was significantly higher than in saliva and plasma of the controls. The 8-OHdG concentration in non-simulated and stimulated saliva as well as plasma of obese teenagers was considerably higher than in their overweight peers (43% $p = 0.001$; 38% $p = 0.007$; 34% $p < 0.001$) (Figure 5).

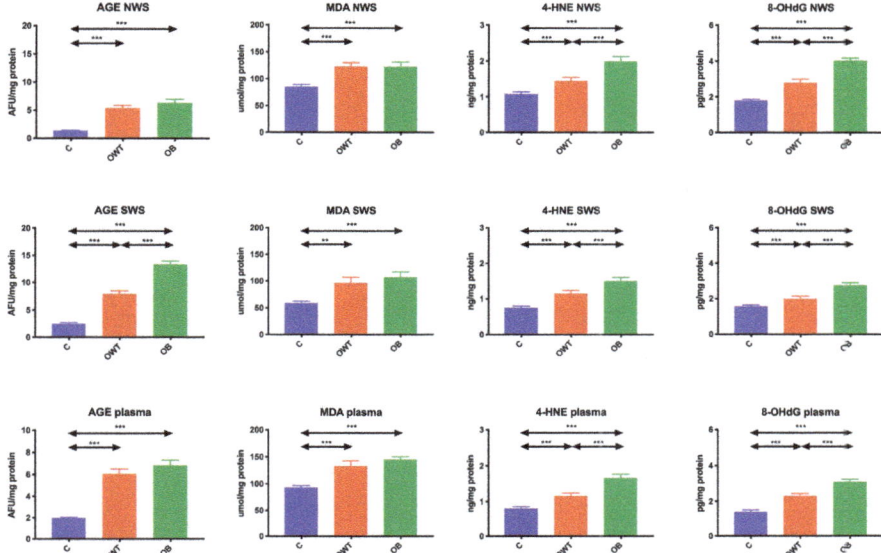

Figure 5. Protein, lipid, and DNA oxidation products in overweight and obese adolescents as well as healthy controls. AGE- advanced glycation end products, C- control, MDA- malondialdehyde, NWS- non-stimulated whole saliva, OB- obese, OWT- overweight, SWS- stimulated whole saliva, 4-HNE- 4-hydroxynoneal protein adduct, 8-OHdG- 8-hydroxy-D-guanosine. Differences statistically significant at: ** $p < 0.005$, *** $p < 0.0005$.

3.6. ROC Analysis

The diagnostic utility of salivary redox parameters to differentiate children who are overweight from those who are obese is presented in Table 3. For this purpose, ROC curves were generated, and then the area under the curve (AUC) was calculated. Optimal cut-off values were determined for each parameter that ensured high sensitivity with high specificity. The maximum AUC value, from 0 to 1, is a parameter that determines the discriminatory power of the test.

Particular attention should be paid to SOD, CAT, TOS and OSI in NWS, GSH and AGE in SWS, and CAT in erythrocytes—the AUC of which is close to 1.0, which differentiates overweight adolescents from obese ones (Figure 6).

Table 3. Receiver operating characteristic (ROC) analysis to differentiate between overweight and obese children.

Parameter	NWS							SWS							Plasma/Erythrocytes					
	AUC	95% Confidence Interval	p Value	Cut-Off	Sensitivity (%)	Specificity (%)		AUC	95% Confidence Interval	p Value	Cut-Off	Sensitivity (%)	Specificity (%)		AUC	95% Confidence Interval	p Value	Cut-Off	Sensitivity (%)	Specificity (%)
Antioxidants																				
SOD (mU/mg protein)	0.7775	0.6222–0.9328	0.0027	>2.469	53.13	63.96		0.615	0.4360–0.7940	0.2134	>4.536	29.93	43.29		0.5325	0.3490–0.7160	0.7251	>0.2348	38.66	38.66
CAT (nmol H$_2$O$_2$/min/mg protein)	0.8875	0.7711–1.000	<0.0001	>0.5747	63.96	69.90		0.6675	0.4954–0.8396	0.0699	>0.5692	43.29	48.10		0.795	0.6515–0.9385	0.0014	<0.6559	53.13	53.13
Px/GPx (mU/mg protein)	0.6575	0.4818–0.8332	0.0884	<0.4494	43.29	38.66		0.5525	0.3675–0.7375	0.57	<0.6815	38.66	34.21		0.5	0.3167–0.6833	>0.9999	>0.3117	34.21	29.93
GSH (µg/mg protein)	0.7	0.5359–0.8641	0.0305	<0.3304	53.1	43.29		0.7925	0.6531–0.9319	0.0016	<0.5908	53.13	48.10		0.5875	0.4058–0.7692	0.3438	<2.823	43.29	34.21
UA (ng/mg protein)	0.67	0.5018–0.8382	0.0659	>0.8843	48.10	34.21		0.5075	0.3247–0.6903	0.9353	>3.912	29.93	29.93		0.6125	0.4345–0.7905	0.2235	>9.354	38.66	43.29
Redox Status																				
TAC (Trolox µmol/mg protein)	0.52	0.3370–0.7030	0.8287	>1.018	34.21	29.93		0.5175	0.3348–0.7002	0.8498	>1.202	29.93	38.66		0.5425	0.3511–0.7339	0.6456	>1.143	34.21	38.66
TOS (nmol H$_2$O$_2$ Equiv/mg protein)	0.9325	0.8344–1.000	<0.0001	>20.77	90	100		0.7425	0.5847–0.9003	0.0087	>45.71	70	80		0.55	0.3685–0.7315	0.5885	<14.48	34.21	29.93
OSI (TOS/TAC ratio)	0.7875	0.6377–0.9373	0.0019	>20.12	80	75		0.655	0.4836–0.8264	0.0935	>38.18	65	60		0.5525	0.3664–0.7386	0.57	<12.63	43.29	34.21
Oxidative Damage																				
AGE (AFU/mg protein)	0.5825	0.3937–0.7713	0.372	>6.116	38.66	48.10		0.9325	0.8547–1.000	<0.0001	>10.24	69.90	69.90		0.6175	0.4395–0.7955	0.2036	>6.360	38.66	38.66
MDA (µmol/mg protein)	0.5325	0.3480–0.7170	0.7251	>127.4	38.66	38.66		0.565	0.3828–0.7472	0.4819	>98.43	43.29	34.21		0.6625	0.4817–0.8433	0.1787	>143.0	53.13	48.10
4-HNE (ng/mg protein)	0.7625	0.6138–0.9112	0.0045	>1.787	65	70		0.705	0.5400–0.8700	0.0265	>1.268	70	70		0.81	0.6730–0.9470	0.0008	>1.386	75	80
8-OHdG (pg/mg protein)	0.8625	0.7452–0.9798	<0.0001	<3.440	80	80		0.795	0.6501–0.9399	0.0014	<2.226	75	80		0.8075	0.6761–0.9389	0.0009	>2.690	65	70

AGE- advanced glycation end products, CAT- catalase, GSH- reduced glutathione, MDA- malondialdehyde, NWS- non-stimulated whole saliva, OSI- oxidative stress index, Px- salivary peroxidase, SOD- superoxide dismutase, SWS- stimulated whole saliva, TAC- total antioxidant capacity, TOS- total oxidative status, UA- uric acid, 4-HNE- 4-hydroxynoneal protein adduct, 8-OHdG- 8-hydroxy-D-guanosine.

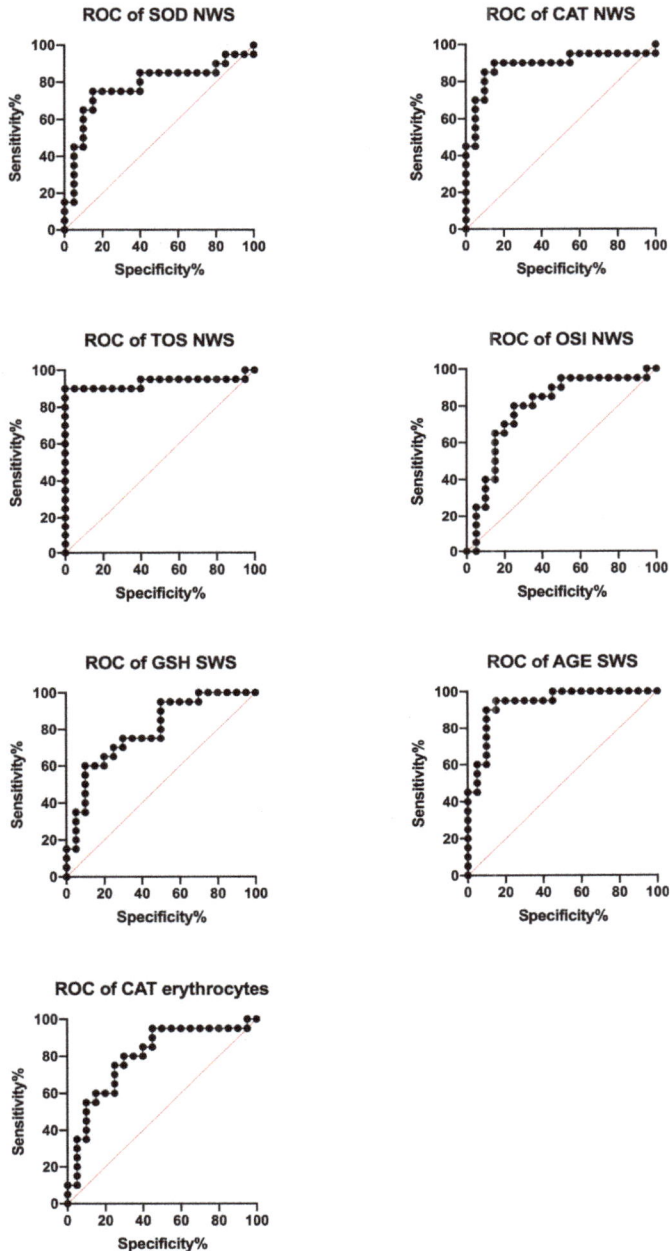

Figure 6. Area under the curve (AUC) of selected redox biomarkers in overweight and obese children. AGE- advanced glycation end products, CAT- catalase, GSH- reduced glutathione, NWS- non-stimulated whole saliva, OSI- oxidative stress index, SOD- superoxide dismutase, SWS- stimulated whole saliva, TOS- total oxidative status, UA- uric acid, 4-HNE- 4-hydroxynoneal protein adduct,.

3.7. Correlations

We showed a positive correlation between erythrocyte and salivary CAT and TAC in overweight and obese adolescents. We also demonstrated a positive correlation between UA content in plasma and non-stimulated/stimulated saliva of the study group patients (Figure 7B). However, we did not observe a saliva–blood correlation of UA in healthy children and adolescents (Figure 7A).

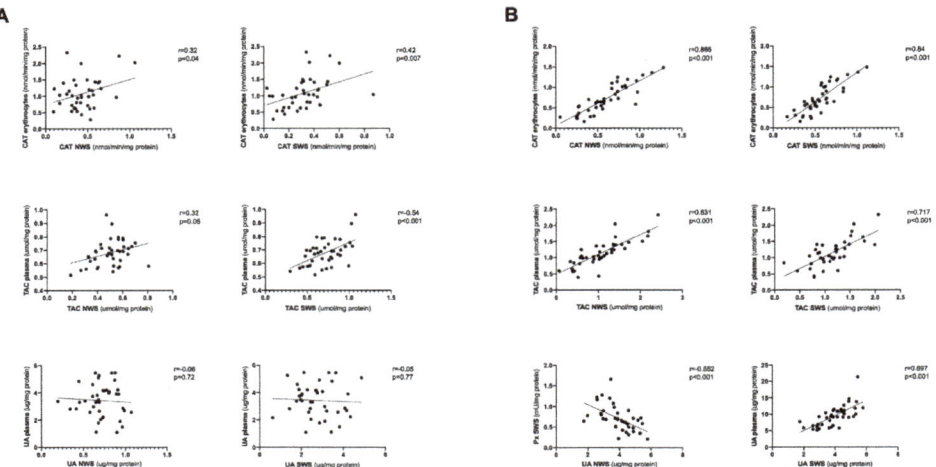

Figure 7. Saliva–blood correlations of the analyzed redox biomarkers in healthy controls (**A**) as well as overweight and obese adolescents (**B**). CAT- catalase, NWS- non-stimulated whole saliva, SWS- stimulated whole saliva, TAC- total antioxidant capacity, UA- uric acid.

Correlations between BMI and salivary redox biomarkers and presented in Figures 8 and 9. Interestingly, BMI correlates with most salivary antioxidants and oxidative damage products but only in the study group.

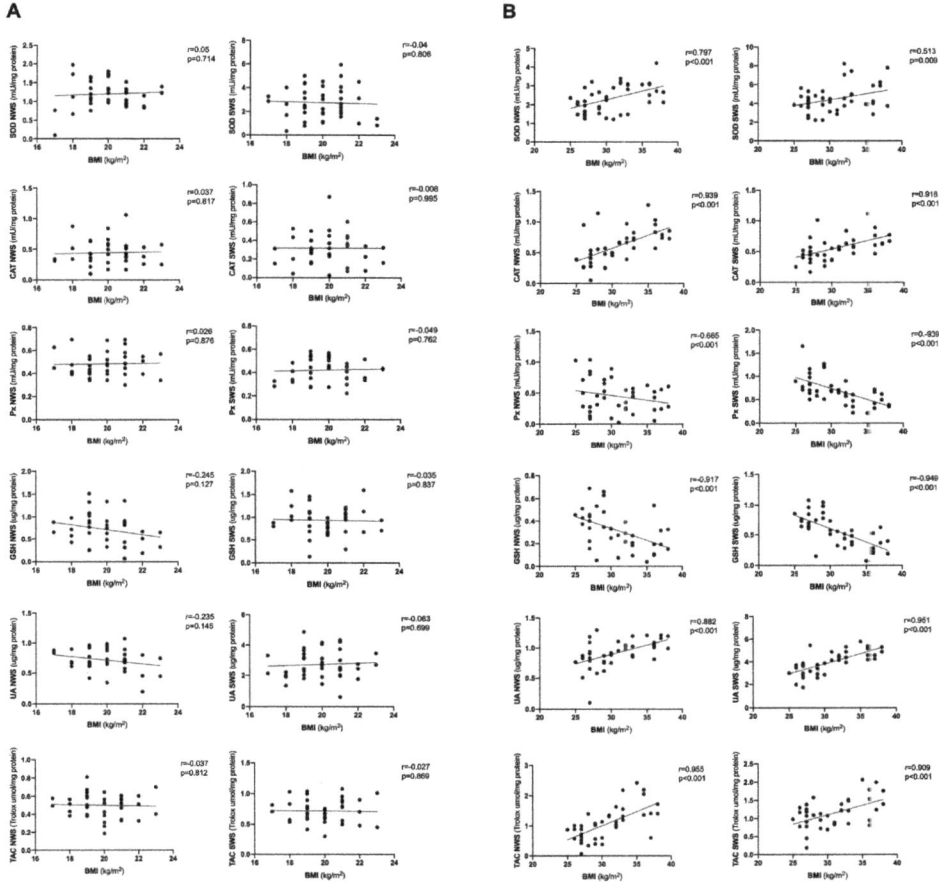

Figure 8. Correlations between BMI and salivary antioxidants in healthy children (**A**) as well as overweight and obese adolescents (**B**). BMI- body mass index, CAT- catalase, GSH- reduced glutathione, NWS- non-stimulated whole saliva, Px- salivary peroxidase, SOD- superoxide dismutase, SWS- stimulated whole saliva, TAC- total antioxidant capacity, UA- uric acid.

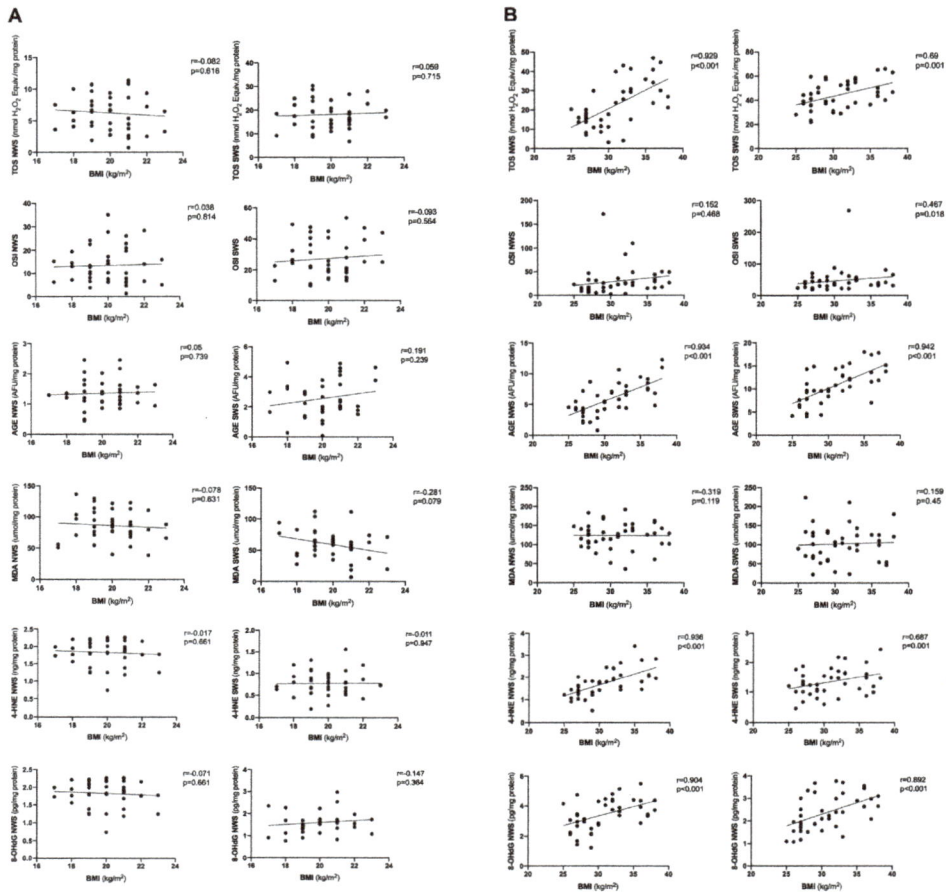

Figure 9. Correlations between BMI and salivary oxidative damage in healthy children (**A**) as well as overweight and obese adolescents (**B**). BMI- body mass index, AGE- advanced glycation end products, MDA- malondialdehyde, NWS- non-stimulated whole saliva, OSI- oxidative stress index, SWS- stimulated whole saliva, TOS- total oxidative status, 4-HNE- 4-hydroxynoneal protein adduct, 8-OHdG- 8-hydroxy-D-guanosine.

4. Discussion

This publication is the first to analyze redox balance in the saliva of overweight and obese adolescents. Generally, we demonstrated disturbances in the activity/concentration of antioxidants as well as oxidative stress in non-stimulated and stimulated saliva of both examined groups compared to their peers with normal body weight, with a higher intensity of oxidative modifications in the saliva of obese adolescents.

Excessive body weight is characterized by chronic (low-grade) inflammation with permanently elevated OS. It has been demonstrated that adipose tissue induces the synthesis of proinflammatory cytokines, such as TNFα, IL-1 and IL-6, which increase the generation of ROS and nitrogen radicals by macrophages and monocytes. ROS production promotes inflammation and expression of molecules as well as growth factors by redox-sensitive transcription factors, mainly NF-κB and the NADPH oxidase pathway [33,34]. The inefficiency of antioxidant systems, observed in the plasma of obese individuals [16], entails oxidative damage to cellular components and development of obesity-related complications.

It has been shown that obesity results in the dysfunction of salivary glands as well as changes in salivary flow and composition [15–17,35]. As saliva is essential for maintaining appropriate functions of the body, such as swallowing, chewing, carbohydrate digestion, healing of the oral mucosa and tooth enamel remineralization, it is not surprising that excessive body weight increases the risk of gingivitis [36], periodontitis [37], caries [38,39] and inflammatory changes in the oral cavity mucosa [40]. Recently, a significant influence of OS has been increasingly emphasized in explaining the pathogenesis of salivary gland lesions in the course of overweight/obesity in adults [16,17,41]. To the best of our knowledge, there have been no studies evaluating redox balance in the oral cavity of overweight and obese adolescents.

The study by Brown et al. [42] demonstrated that failure of antioxidant systems is related to the duration of obesity. Considering that our study covered adolescents aged 11 to 18 with relatively short overweight/obesity history (4/4.3 years, respectively, data not shown), it is not surprising that salivary and plasma TAC (the sum of both enzymatic and non-enzymatic antioxidants) as well as the content of enzymatic antioxidants were elevated in both non-stimulated and stimulated saliva of overweight and obese adolescents. Therefore, the higher activity of enzymatic antioxidants may be an expression of a highly effective antioxidant barrier that has not been exhausted in oxidative stress conditions. On the other hand, a significant increase in salivary TAC and enzymatic antioxidants as well as, generally, plasma biomarkers (despite the decline in SOD activity, which we explain further) can be considered as a positive adaptative response to the increased ROS generation (↑TOS in plasma as well as non-stimulated and stimulated saliva of both study groups). It was demonstrated that decreased activity of antioxidant enzymes in erythrocytes, accompanying increased plasma TAC, is likely to result from cell damage due to an inflammatory process and leakage of enzymes into the extracellular space [43]. On the other hand, it may result from the use of enzymes in the process of ROS control, or from inactivation of enzymes by free radicals [44].

Interestingly, we found a significant positive correlation between erythrocyte and salivary CAT and TAC in overweight and obese adolescents, which suggests that these salivary parameters could assess the general antioxidant status of overweight and obese adolescents.

Uric acid constitutes 40% of the antioxidant potential of saliva [45]; however, it has been found that at high concentrations it can induce and intensify oxidative damage [46]. Obesity has been demonstrated to increase UA concentration by reducing its renal secretion and accumulating metabolites for UA production [47], which was confirmed by our study. We observed an increase in uric acid concentration both in plasma and stimulated saliva of overweight and obese adolescents as well as in non-stimulated saliva of the latter. The negative correlation between the concentrations of UA and protein in non-stimulated saliva of overweight and obese adolescents, as well as the negative correlation between UA content and Px activity in stimulated saliva, suggest that in both groups UA shifts salivary redox balance towards oxidation and does not oxidize hydroxyl or peroxyl radicals, preventing OS. Moreover, we demonstrated a positive correlation between UA levels in plasma and stimulated saliva of overweight and obese subjects. Considering that plasma UA is a strong predictor of future development of type 2 diabetes [48], measurements of salivary UA may be useful in assessing the risk of this disease.

Although changes in the activity/concentration of antioxidants or ROS concentration may suggest redox imbalance, they are not sufficient to determine the existence and extent of OS. The most reliable determinants of oxidative stress are increased concentrations of oxidative damage products [49,50]. There are numerous markers of oxidative damage to biomolecules; in our study, we assessed 4-HNE protein adducts, MDA, AGE and 8-OHdG. These are only few selected markers, which should be taken into account when interpreting the presented results. The use of other OS indicators could change our observations and conclusions.

Our research showed, however, that the overproduction of free radicals exceeds the capabilities of antioxidant systems of the examined adolescents at the central level as well as in both salivary glands, which was observed as increased concentration of oxidative modification products in plasma and non-stimulated as well as stimulated saliva. It should be noted that intensified oxidative modifications reveal a certain tendency (AGE and MDA in plasma and non-stimulated saliva; MDA in stimulated saliva) or are significantly higher (4-HNE, 8-OHdG in plasma and stimulated and non-stimulated saliva, and AGE in stimulated saliva) in obese adolescents compared to their overweight peers. The obtained results prove that oxidative damage occurred in the salivary glands of overweight adolescents, and was more severe in obese subjects. We noted a significant increase of TOS in non-stimulated and stimulated saliva in obese adolescents compared to the overweight group, but observed no such dependence for TAC and antioxidant enzymes (except CAT in non-stimulated saliva). In our opinion, this is a worrying phenomenon and may be evidence of the beginning of subclinical inefficiency of antioxidant mechanisms, leading to the boost of oxidative damage to the salivary glands of obese adolescents.

We demonstrated that in both non-stimulated and stimulated saliva of overweight and obese patients, GSH levels were significantly decreased and considerably lower in the stimulated saliva of patients with obesity compared to overweight ones. Our results suggest that, GSH is the first to be used up, and perhaps forms the first line of defense against free radicals, which can be easily explained. The main function of GSH is maintaining thiol groups of proteins in a reduced state, which is often necessary for preserving the functional activity of these proteins. It has been shown that the most probable primary object of ROS attack is proteins, and, according to this theory, fatty and nucleic acids are protected by proteins and therefore undergo oxidation at a later stage [51]. A mediator of biomolecule damage in cells is the hydroxyl radical (OH·) [52]. It was shown that the percentage share of primary substrates of the OH· reaction is 75% proteins, 21% lipids, and 4% DNA, which is related to the specificity of the mechanism of OH· radical production in the Fenton reaction [52].

It is worth mentioning that the stimulation of saliva secretion activates parotid glands, while at rest the main source of saliva is the submandibular glands. Therefore, it was assumed that any disturbances in secretion/composition of non-stimulated saliva reflects disturbances of the submandibular gland function, and disturbed secretion/composition of stimulated saliva indicates disturbed activity of parotid glands [53].

The ability of salivary glands of overweight and obese adolescents to secrete saliva at rest was similar to the results of their peers of normal weight. Protein secretion by submandibular glands of the examined adolescents also did not differ from the control group of normal weight. In relation to the stimulated salivary flow, overweight and obese subjects showed reduced salivary secretion compared to the control group, which is consistent with the results of Modéer et al. [38]. Moreover, the dysfunction of parotid glands intensified with the increase in BMI, as obese adolescents produce significantly less stimulated saliva than their overweight peers, and in 8 obese individuals we recorded the salivary flow value of 0.7 mL/min, which is classified as hyposalivation. Modéer et al. [38] claimed that BMI SDS may be a potential factor to exclude subjects with reduced flow of stimulated saliva. Protein concentration in SWS of overweight and obese adolescents was also reduced compared to the controls. The decrease in stimulated saliva secretion and protein concentration is most probably caused by steatosis of the parotid (but not submandibular) glands observed in obese patients, which decreases the number of secretory units (acini and ducts) [54,55]. It can also be assumed that obesity-related inflammatory milieu (up-regulation of proinflammatory cytokines, ROS), similarly to Sjögren's syndrome [56], activates metalloproteinases, thus disrupting the stromal tissue. This phenomenon may disturb the neurotransmission between the residual neural network and residual secretory units, as well as inhibit the response of follicular cells [57,58].

Our study showed reduced salivary production and enhanced oxidative stress in overweight and obese teenagers. However, in obese children, alterations in salivary gland function are more severe than those who are overweight. This is also reflected in the redox status of saliva (greater disturbances in the antioxidant barrier) as well as higher severity of oxidative damage in children with obesity vs. overweight.

5. Conclusions

Obese and overweight adolescents present impaired systemic and salivary oxidative status in contrast to their normal weight peers.

Both parotid and submandibular salivary glands lose the ability to maintain redox balance at the level observed in the control group, which was shown by an increased level of oxidized biomolecules. However, redox equilibrium in our study was more disturbed in the saliva and plasma of obese adolescents compared to overweight subjects.

Excess of adipose tissue and deficiency of GSH are the main factors responsible for oxidative damage to the salivary glands.

Dysfunction of parotid glands in relation to salivary secretion deepens with the increase of BMI. Dysfunction of mechanisms responsible for protein synthesis/secretion observed at the overweight stage does not worsen with the increase of body weight in adolescents.

Determinations of salivary CAT and TAC could be used to assess the central antioxidant status of overweight and obese adolescents.

Author Contributions: Conceptualization, A.Z., M.M.; Data curation, A.Z. and M.M.;A.K., S.Z., Formal analysis, A.Z. and M.M. A.K., S.Z.; Funding acquisition, A.Z.; Investigation, A.Z. and M.M.; Methodology, A.Z., M.M.; Material collection: A.K., K.F., M.S., P.K-S., Supervision, A.Z., K.T-J., A.W.; Validation, A.Z. and M.M.; Visualization, A.Z. and M.M.; Writing—original draft, A.Z. and M.M.; Writing—review and editing, A.Z. and M.M. All authors have read and agreed to the published version of the manuscript.

Funding: This work was supported by grants from the Medical University of Bialystok, Poland (grant numbers: SUB/1/DN/20/002/1209; SUB/1/DN/20/002/3330).

Conflicts of Interest: The authors declare no conflict of interest.

References

1. Marseglia, L.; Manti, S.; D'Angelo, G.; Nicotera, A.; Parisi, E.; Di Rosa, G.; Gitto, E.; Arrigo, T. Oxidative stress in obesity: A critical component in human diseases. *Int. J. Mol. Sci.* **2014**, *16*, 378–400. [CrossRef]
2. Rowicka, G.; Dylag, H.; Ambroszkiewicz, J.; Riahi, A.; Weker, H.; Chelchowska, M. Total Oxidant and Antioxidant Status in Prepubertal Children with Obesity. *Oxid. Med. Cell. Longev.* **2017**. [CrossRef] [PubMed]
3. Matczuk, J.; Zalewska, A.; Łukaszuk, B.; Knaś, M.; Maciejczyk, M.; Grabowska, M.; Ziembicka, D.M.; Waszkiel, D.; Chabowski, A.; Żendzian-Piotrowska, M.; et al. Insulin resistance and obesity affect lipid profile in the salivary glands. *J. Diabetes Res.* **2016**. [CrossRef] [PubMed]
4. WHO. Global Database on Body Mass Index. Available online: http://www.who.int/bmi (accessed on 16 January 2020).
5. Freedman, D.S.; Khan, L.K.; Serdula, M.K.; Dietz, W.H.; Srinivasan, S.R.; Berenson, G.S. The relation of childhood BMI to adult adiposity: The Bogalusa Heart Study. *Pediatrics* **2005**, *115*, 22–27. [CrossRef] [PubMed]
6. Knaś, M.; Maciejczyk, M.; Waszkiel, D.; Zalewska, A. Oxidative stress and salivary antioxidants. *Dent. Med. Probl.* **2013**, *50*, 461–466.
7. Holven, K.B.; Ulven, S.M.; Bogsrud, M.P. Hyperlipidemia and cardiovascular disease with focus on familial hypercholesterolemia. *Curr. Opin. Lipidol.* **2017**, *28*, 445–447. [CrossRef]
8. Kurek, K.; Miklosz, A.; Lukaszuk, B.; Chabowski, A.; Gorski, J.; Zendzian-Piotrowska, M. Inhibition of Ceramide De Novo Synthesis Ameliorates Diet Induced Skeletal Muscles Insulin Resistance. *J. Diabetes Res.* **2015**. [CrossRef]
9. Outon, S.; Galceran, I.; Pascual, J.; Oliveras, A. Central blood pressure in morbid obesity and after bariatric surgery. *Nefrologia* **2019**. [CrossRef]
10. Greig, F.; Hyman, S.; Wallach, E.; Hildebrandt, T.; Rapaport, R. Which obese youth are at increased risk for type 2 diabetes? Latent class analysis and comparison with diabetic youth. *Pediatr. Diabetes* **2012**, *13*, 181–188. [CrossRef]

11. Sanchez, A.; Furberg, H.; Kuo, F.; Vuong, L.; Ged, Y.; Patil, S.; Ostrovnaya, I.; Petruzella, S.; Reising, A.; Patel, P.; et al. Transcriptomic signatures related to the obesity paradox in patients with clear cell renal cell carcinoma: A cohort study. *Lancet Oncol.* **2019**. [CrossRef]
12. Gerdin, E.W.; Angbratt, M.; Aronsson, K.; Eriksson, E.; Johansson, I. Dental caries and body mass index by socio-economic status in Swedish children. *Commun. Dent. Oral. Epidemiol.* **2008**, *36*, 459–465. [CrossRef] [PubMed]
13. Willerhausen, B.; Blettner, M.; Kasaj, A.; Hohenfellner, K. Association between body mass index and dental health in 1,290 children of elementary schools in a German city. *Clin. Oral. Invesitg.* **2007**, *11*, 195–200. [CrossRef]
14. Zeigler, C.C.; Persson, G.R.; Wondimu, B.; Marcus, C.; Sobko, T.; Modèer, T. Microbiota in the oral subgingival biofilm is associated with obesity in adolescence. *Obesity* **2012**, *20*, 157–164. [CrossRef] [PubMed]
15. Chielle, E.O.; Casarin, J.N. Evaluation of salivary oxidative parameters in overweight and obese young adults. *Arch. Epidemiol. Metab.* **2017**, *61*, 152–159. [CrossRef] [PubMed]
16. Knaś, M.; Maciejczyk, M.; Sawicka, K.; Hady Razak, H.; Niczyporuk, M.; Ładny, J.R.; Matczuk, J.; Waszkiel, D.; Żendzian-Piotrowska, M.; Zalewska, A. Impact of morbid obesity and bariatric surgery on antioxidant/oxidant balance of the unstimulated and stimulated saliva. *J. Oral. Pathol. Med.* **2016**, *45*, 455–464. [CrossRef]
17. Fejfer, K.; Buczko, P.; Niczyporuk, M.; Ładny, J.R.; Hady, R.H.; Knaś, M.; Waszkiel, D.; Klimiuk, A.; Zalewska, A.; Maciejczyk, M. Oxidative Modicication of biomolecules in the nonstiumulated and stimulated saliva of patients with morbid obesity treated with bariatric surgery. *BioMed Res. Int.* **2017**. [CrossRef]
18. Narotzki, B.; Reznick, A.Z.; Mitki, T.; Aizenbud, D.; Levy, Y. Enhanced cardiovascular risk and altered oxidative status in elders with moderate excessive body fat. *Rejuvenation Res.* **2014**, *17*, 334–340. [CrossRef]
19. Cole, T.J.; Green, P.J. Smoothing reference centile curves: The LMS method and penalized likelihood. *Stat. Med.* **1992**, *11*, 1305–1319. [CrossRef]
20. WHO. *WHO Child Growth Standards: Length/Height-for-Age, Weight-for-Age, Weight-for-Length, Weight-for-Height and Body Mass Index-Forage: Methods and Development*; WHO: Genewa, Switzerland, 2006.
21. De Onis, M.; Lobstein, T. Defining obesity risk status in the general childhood population: Which cut-offs should we use? *Int. J. Pediatr. Obese.* **2010**, *5*, 458–460. [CrossRef]
22. Mansson-Rahemtulla, B.; Baldone, D.C.; Pruitt, K.M.; Rahemtulla, F. Specific assays for peroxidases in human saliva. *Arch. Oral. Biol.* **1986**, *31*, 661–668. [CrossRef]
23. Aebi, H. Catalase in vitro. *Methods Enzymol.* **1984**, *105*, 121–126. [PubMed]
24. Misra, H.P.; Fridovich, I. The role of superoxide anion in the autoxidation of epinephrine and a simple assay for superoxide dismutase. *J. Biol. Chem.* **1972**, *247*, 3170–3175. [PubMed]
25. Griffith, O.W. Determination of glutathione and glutathione disulfide using glutathione reductase and 2-vinylpyridine. *Anal. Biochem.* **1980**, *106*, 207–212. [CrossRef]
26. Erel, O. A novel automated direct measurement method for total antioxidant capacity using a new generation, more stable ABTS radical cation. *Clin. Biochem.* **2004**, *37*, 227–285. [CrossRef] [PubMed]
27. Erel, O. A new automated colorimetric method for measuring total oxidant status. *Clin. Biochem.* **2005**, *38*, 1103–1111. [CrossRef]
28. Kołodziej, U.; Maciejczyk, M.; Niklińska, W.; Waszkiel, D.; Żendzian-Piotrowska, M.; Żukowski, P.; Zalewska, A. Chronic high-protein diet induces oxidative stress and alters the salivary gland function in rats. *Arch. Oral. Biol.* **2017**, *84*, 6–12. [CrossRef]
29. Abuelo, A.; Hernandez, J.; Benedito, J.L.; Castillo, C. Oxidative stress index (OSI) as a new tool to assess redox status in dairy cattle during transition period. *Animal* **2013**, *7*, 1374–1378. [CrossRef]
30. Kalousová, M.; Skrha, J.; Zima, T. Advanced glycation end-products and advanced oxidation protein products in patients with diabetes mellitus. *Physiol. Res.* **2002**, *51*, 597–604.
31. Maciejczyk, M.; Zalewska, A.; Ladny, J.R. Salivary Antioxidant Barrier, Redox Status, and Oxidative Damage to Proteins and Lipids in Healthy Children, Adults, and the Elderly. *Oxid. Med. Cell. Longev.* **2019**. [CrossRef]
32. Buege, J.A.; Aust, S.D. Microsomal lipid peroxidation. *Methods Enzymol.* **1978**, *52*, 302–310.
33. Farhangi, M.A.; Mesgari-Abbasi, M.; Hajiluian, G.; Nameni, G.; Shahabi, P. Adipose Tissue Inflammation and Oxidative Stress: The Ameliorative Effects of Vitamin D. *Inflammation* **2017**, *40*, 1688–1697. [CrossRef] [PubMed]

34. Alcala, M.; Calderon-Dominguez, M.; Bustos, E.; Ramos, P.; Casals, N.; Serra, D.; Viana, M.; Herrero, L. Increased inflammation, oxidative stress and mitochondrial respiration in brown adipose tissue from obese mice. *Sci. Rep.* **2017**. [CrossRef] [PubMed]
35. Pannunzio, E.; Silverio Amancio, O.M.; de Souza Vitalle, M.S.; Nesadal de Souza, D.; Medeiros Mendes, F.; Nicolau, J. Analysis of the stimulated whole saliva in overweight and obese children. *Rev. Assoc. Med. Bras.* **2010**, *56*, 32–36. [CrossRef] [PubMed]
36. Zhao, B.; Jin, C.; Li, L.; Wang, Y. Increased Expression of TNF-alpha Occurs Before the Development of Periodontitis Among Obese Chinese Children: A Potential Marker for Prediction and Prevention of Periodontitis. *Oral. Health Prev. Dent.* **2016**, *14*, 71–75. [CrossRef]
37. Scorzetti, L.; Marcattili, D.; Pasini, M.; Mattei, A.; Marchetti, E.; Marzo, G. Association between obesity and periodontal disease in children. *Eur. J. Pediatr. Dent.* **2013**, *14*, 181–184.
38. Modeer, T.; Blomberg, C.C.; Wondimu, B.; Julihn, A.; Marcus, C. Association between obesity, flow rate of whole saliva, and dental caries in adolescents. *Obesity* **2010**, *18*, 2367–2373. [CrossRef]
39. Fadel, H.T.; Pliaki, A.; Gronowitz, E.; Mårild, S.; Ramberg, P.; Dahlèn, G.; Yucel-Lindberg, T.; Heijl, L.; Birkhed, D. Clinical and biological indicators of dental caries and periodontal disease in adolescents with or without obesity. *Clin. Oral. Investig.* **2014**, *18*, 359–368. [CrossRef]
40. Patrascu, V.; Giurca, C.; Ciurea, R.N.; Georgescu, C.C.; Ciurea, M.E. Ulcerated necrobiosis lipoidica to a teenager with diabetes mellitus and obesity. *Rom. J. Morphol. Embryol.* **2014**, *55*, 171–176.
41. Dursun, E.; Akalin, F.A.; Genc, T.; Cinar, N.; Erel, O.; Yildiz, B.O. Oxidative stress and periodontal disease in obesity. *Medicine* **2016**, *95*, e3136. [CrossRef]
42. Brown, L.A.; Kerr, C.J.; Whiting, P.; Finer, N.; McEneny, J.; Ashton, T. Oxidant stress in healthy normal-weight, overweight, and obese individuals. *Obesity* **2009**, *17*, 460–466. [CrossRef]
43. Goth, L.; Lenkey, A.; Bigler, W.N. Blood catalase deficiency and diabetes in Hungary. *Diabetes Care* **2001**, *24*, 1839–1840. [CrossRef] [PubMed]
44. Zalewska, A.; Knaś, M.; Waszkiewicz, N.; Klimiuk, A.; Litwin, K.; Sierakowski, S.; Waszkiel, D Salivary antioxidants in patients with systemic sclerosis. *J. Oral. Pathol. Med.* **2014**, *43*, 61–68. [CrossRef] [PubMed]
45. Zalewska, A.; Knaś, M.; Żendzian-Piotrowska, M.; Waszkiewicz, N.; Szulimowska, J.; Prokopiuk, S.; Waszkiel, D.; Car, H. Antioxidant profile of salivary glands in high fat diet- induced insulin resistance rats. *Oral. Dis.* **2014**, *20*, 560–566. [CrossRef] [PubMed]
46. Al-Rawi, N.H. Oxidative stress, antioxidant status and lipid profile in the saliva of type 2 diabetics. *Diabetes Vasc. Dis. Res.* **2011**, *8*, 22–28. [CrossRef]
47. Yuan, H.; Yang, X.; Shi, X.; Tian, R.; Zhao, Z. Association of serum uric acid with different levels of glucose and related factors. *Chin. Med. J.* **2011**, *124*, 1443–1448. [PubMed]
48. Wang, Z.N.; Li, P.; Jiang, R.H.; Li, L.; Li, X.; Li, L.; Liu, C.; Tian, C.L. The association between serum uric acid and metabolic syndrome among adolescents in northeast China. *Int. J. Clin. Exp. Med.* **2015**, *8*, 21122–21129.
49. Lushchak, V.I. Free radicals, reactive oxygen species, oxidative stress and its classification. *Chem. Biol. Interact.* **2014**, *224*, 164–175. [CrossRef]
50. Lushchak, V.I. Classification of oxidative stress based on its intensity. *Exp. Clin. Sci.* **2014**, *13*, 922–937.
51. Adamczyk-Sowa, M.; Bieszczad-Bedrejczuk, E.; Galiniak, S.; Rozmilowska, I.; Czyzewski, D.; Bartosz, G.; Sadowska-Bartosz, I. Oxidative modifications of blood serum proteins in myasthenia gravis. *J. Neuroimmunol.* **2017**, *305*, 145–153. [CrossRef]
52. Gębicki, J.M.; Bartosz, G. Rola białek jako przekaźników uszkodzeń indukowanych przez reaktywne formy tlenu in vivo. *Postepy Biochem.* **2010**, *56*, 115–123.
53. Choromańska, M.; Klimiuk, A.; Kostecka-Sochoń, P.; Wilczyńska, K.; Kwiatkowski, M.; Okuniewska, N.; Waszkiewicz, N.; Zalewska, A.; Maciejczyk, M. Antioxidant defence, oxidative stress and oxidative damage in saliva, plasma and erythrocytes of dementia patients. Can salivary AGE be a marker of dementia? *Int. J. Mol. Sci.* **2017**, *18*, 2205. [CrossRef] [PubMed]
54. Bozzato, A.; Burger, P.; Zenk, J.; Ulter, W.; Iro, H. Salivary gland biometry in female patients with eating disorders. *Eur. Arch. Oto-Rhino-Laryngol.* **2008**, *265*, 1095–1102. [CrossRef]
55. Heo, M.S.; Lee, S.C.; Lee, S.S.; Choi, H.M.; Choi, S.C.; Park, T.W. Quantitative analysis of normal major salivary glands using computed tomography. *Oral Surg. Oral Med. Oral Pathol. Oral Radiol. Endodontol.* **2001**, *92*, 240–244. [CrossRef] [PubMed]

56. Sekiguchi, M.; Iwasaki, T.; Kitano, M.; Kuno, H.; Hashimoto, N.; Kawahito, Y.; Azuma, M.; Hla, T.; Sano, H. Role of sphingosine 1-phosphate in the pathogenesis of Sjögren's syndrome. *J. Immunol.* **2008**, *180*, 1921–1928. [CrossRef]
57. Uemura, T.; Suzuki, T.; Saiki, R.; Dohmae, N.; Ito, S.; Takahashi, H.; Toida, T.; Kashiwagi, K.; Igarashi, K. Activation of MMP-9 activity by acrolein in saliva from patients with primary Sjögren's syndrome and its mechanism. *Int. J. Biochem. Cell Biol.* **2017**, *88*, 84–91. [CrossRef] [PubMed]
58. Norheim, K.B.; Jonsson, G.; Harboe, E.; Hanasand, M.; Goransson, L.; Omdal, R. Oxidative stress, as measured by protein oxidation, is increased in primary Sjögren's syndrome. *Free Radic. Res.* **2012**, *46*, 141–146. [CrossRef] [PubMed]

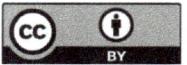

© 2020 by the authors. Licensee MDPI, Basel, Switzerland. This article is an open access article distributed under the terms and conditions of the Creative Commons Attribution (CC BY) license (http://creativecommons.org/licenses/by/4.0/).

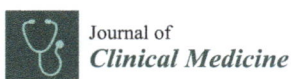

Article

Salivary Cytokine Biomarker Concentrations in Relation to Obesity and Periodontitis

Sanna Syrjäläinen [1], Ulvi Kahraman Gursoy [1,*], Mervi Gursoy [1], Pirkko Pussinen [2], Milla Pietiäinen [2], Antti Jula [3], Veikko Salomaa [3], Pekka Jousilahti [3] and Eija Könönen [1,4]

1. Periodontology, Institute of Dentistry, University of Turku, 20520 Turku, Finland; sanna.syrjalainen@utu.fi (S.S.); mervi.gursoy@utu.fi (M.G.); eija.kononen@utu.fi (E.K.)
2. Oral and Maxillofacial Diseases, University of Helsinki, 00014 Helsinki, Finland; pirkko.pussinen@helsinki.fi (P.P.); milla.pietiainen@helsinki.fi (M.P.)
3. Finnish Institute for Health and Welfare, 00271 Helsinki, Finland; antti.jula@thl.fi (A.J.); veikko.salomaa@thl.fi (V.S.); pekka.jousilahti@thl.fi (P.J.)
4. Oral Health Care, Welfare Division, City of Turku, 20101 Turku, Finland
* Correspondence: ulvi.gursoy@utu.fi; Tel.: +358-50-514-8132

Received: 25 November 2019; Accepted: 3 December 2019; Published: 5 December 2019

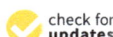

Abstract: Systemic low-grade inflammation is associated with obesity. Our aim was to examine the association between obesity and salivary biomarkers of periodontitis. Salivary interleukin (IL)-1-receptor antagonist (IL-1Ra), IL-6, IL-8, IL-10, and tumor necrosis factor (TNF)-α concentrations were measured from 287 non-diabetic obese (body mass index (BMI) of >35 kg/m^2) individuals and 293 normal-weight (BMI of 18.5–25 kg/m^2) controls. Periodontal status was defined according to a diagnostic cumulative risk score (CRS) to calculate the risk of having periodontitis (CRS I, low risk; CRS II, medium risk; CRS III, high risk). In the whole population, and especially in smokers, higher IL-8 and lower IL-10 concentrations were detected in the obese group compared to the control group, while in non-smoking participants, the obese and control groups did not differ. IL-1Ra and IL-8 concentrations were higher in those with medium or high risk (CRS II and CRS III, $p < 0.001$) of periodontitis, whereas IL-10 and TNF-α concentrations were lower when compared to those with low risk (CRS I). In multivariate models adjusted for periodontal status, obesity did not associate with any salivary cytokine concentration. In conclusion, salivary cytokine biomarkers are not independently associated with obesity and concentrations are dependent on periodontal status.

Keywords: obesity; periodontitis; cytokine; inflammation; saliva

1. Introduction

Obesity is an increasing health problem in developed countries and is a major risk factor for diabetes, cancer, and cardiovascular diseases [1]. Obesity is linked to both local and systemic inflammation [2–5]. In obese subjects, there is an elevated release of proinflammatory cytokines into serum derived from either adipocytes, stromal vascular fraction cells, or immune cells in adipose tissue [3,5,6]. This elevated cytokine release in obese individuals is a reversible condition, since even mild weight loss can reduce serum cytokine levels [7].

There is substantial evidence showing a positive association between obesity or weight gain and periodontitis [8–11]. The underlying mechanisms explaining this association are not completely elucidated, but one proposed mechanism is that the low-grade systemic inflammation related to obesity could expose obese people to infectious diseases [3,4,12]. Pathogenic bacterial biofilms at the gingival margin trigger the initiation of inflammatory processes in periodontal tissues, including the production of chemokines and proinflammatory cytokines [13,14]. Inflammatory cytokines in the periodontium are low-molecular weight proteins secreted from both periodontal tissue and immune cells [13]. They are the main regulators of inflammation and tissue destruction in periodontitis [15], and their levels in saliva predict periodontal disease progression and remission [16]. To our knowledge, the association between salivary cytokine concentrations and obesity and periodontitis has not been examined in humans so far.

In the present study, we used a novel diagnostic method, the cumulative risk score (CRS), to detect periodontal disease based on three biomarkers in saliva [17]. CRS combines *Porphyromonas gingivalis*, interleukin (IL)-1β, and matrix metalloproteinase (MMP)-8, and categorizes individuals with low, medium, or high risk of having periodontitis. Our hypothesis is that low-grade inflammation related to obesity affects the cytokine biomarker concentrations in saliva. In this context, our cross-sectional study aimed to examine the relation between obesity and periodontitis-associated salivary cytokine concentrations in smoking and non-smoking individuals.

2. Experimental Section

2.1. Study Population

The study consisted of 580 individuals aged 25–74 (mean 55.3) years. They were participants of the Dietary, Lifestyle, and Genetic determinant of Obesity and Metabolic syndrome (DILGOM) study, which was an extension of the population-based National FINRISK2007 health survey to investigate more specifically the effects of diet, lifestyle, and genetic factors on obesity and metabolic syndrome [18,19]. Of the 5024 individuals who participated in the DILGOM study, 287 severely obese (body mass index (BMI) ≥35 kg/m^2) and 297 normal-weight (BMI 18.5–25 kg/m^2) controls matched for age and smoking status were included. Exclusion criteria for both cases and controls were diabetes, cardiovascular disease, cancer, or medication for hypercholesterolemia. The protocol of the FINRISK2007 survey included questionnaire data on smoking and other health behaviors, socioeconomic background factors, clinical measurements, and venous blood samples. Participants were categorized by their smoking status as current smokers or non-smokers (smokeless for at least the past 6 months). Height was measured to the nearest 0.1 cm and weight to the nearest 0.1 kg.

2.2. Bacterial and Cytokine Measurements from Salivary Samples

Paraffin-stimulated whole saliva samples were collected by expectoration into plastic tubes from the DILGOM study participants. All samples were stored frozen at −70 °C until laboratory analyses. Before analyses, melted samples were gently mixed, and centrifuged at 10,000 × g for 5 min. DNA was isolated from the pellet and used in *P. gingivalis* quantification, while the supernatant was used in cytokine determinations.

Salivary concentrations of IL-1β, IL-1 receptor antagonist (IL-1Ra), IL-6, IL-8, IL-10, tumor necrosis factor alpha (TNF–α), and MMP-8 were analyzed with the flow-cytometric Luminex xMAP technique with commercially available kits by Bio-PlexTM 200 (Bio-Rad Laboratories Incorporation, Santa Rosa, CA, USA).

The amounts of *P. gingivalis* were determined with a quantitative real-time PCR (qPCR) assay as previously described [20] with modifications. Reaction mixtures (total volume 20 μL) contained 2 μL of template DNA, 200 nM primers (Thermo Fisher Scientific, Waltham, MA, USA), and 1 × Universal KAPA SYBR FAST qPCR mastermix (KAPA Biosystems, Wilmington, MA, USA) supplemented with 1 × ROX Low reference dye. qPCR analyses were performed with the Mx3005P Real-Time qPCR System (Stratagene, La Jolla, CA, USA) via the following steps: Initial denaturation at 95 °C for 3 min, followed by 40 cycles of 3 s at 95 °C and 20 s at 60 °C. A dissociation curve was generated from one cycle of 1 min at 95 °C, then lowering the temperature gradually to 60 °C, 30 s at 60 °C, then raising the temperature gradually to 95 °C, and 30 s at 95 °C. The data were analyzed with the Mx3005P Real-Time qPCR System software and the results were presented as genomic equivalents (GE)/mL saliva.

For the standard curve, the whole *P. gingivalis waaA* gene, encoding 3-deoxy-D-manno-oct-2-ulosonic acid (Kdo) transferase, was cloned to pJet1.2/blunt vector (Thermo Fisher Scientific, Waltham, MA, USA). The cloned fragment was PCR-amplified in the reaction containing 500 nM primers (Fwd-ATGCGATTCCTTTTCAG and Rew-CTATTTCATGATTCGGTG), 200 µM dNTPs, Phusion DNA Polymerase (Thermo Fisher Scientific, Waltham, MA, USA) 0.04 U/µL, 1 × Phusion High-Fidelity Buffer, and 10 ng of chromosomal DNA of *P. gingivalis* strain W50. The cycling conditions followed the manufacturer's instructions. The purified PCR fragment was ligated into pJet1.2/blunt vector with CloneJET PCR Cloning Kit (Thermo Fisher Scientific, Waltham, MA, USA) according to the manufacturer's instructions and ligation mixture was transformed into *Escherichia coli* DH5a competent cells. The correct insert was verified by sequencing. The constructed plasmid, pJet1.2/blunt-Pg, was linearized with FastDigest HindIII restriction enzyme (Thermo Fisher Scientific, Waltham, MA, USA) and used for a tenfold dilution series for the qPCR analysis. The plasmid copy number was determined with "DNA Copy Number and Dilution Calculator" (www.thermofisher.com).

2.3. Periodontal Status Assessment Based on Cumulative Risk Score (CRS)

Periodontal status of the study population ($n = 580$) was defined according to CRS as described in detail by Gursoy et al. [17]. Briefly, for calculating CRS, the salivary concentrations of *P. gingivalis*, IL-1β, and MMP-8 were independently divided into tertiles and each participant was categorized to one of the three tertiles according to the level of the biomarker in the saliva. The person's cumulative score was calculated by multiplication of three biomarkers' tertile values. Based on these calculations, the study participants were categorized into three periodontal status groups, as follows: CRS I: low risk; CRS II: medium risk; CRS III: High risk [17,21,22].

2.4. Statistical Analyses

All statistical analyses were conducted using the IBM SPSS Statistic 23.0 software (IBM, Armonk, North Castle, NY, USA). In descriptive statistics, continuous variables were reported as means and standard deviations and the differences between the groups were analyzed by independent *t*-test. Categorical variables were reported as the number of individuals and as percentages. Differences between the groups in categorical variables were analyzed using the chi-square test. Statistical significance was set at a *p*-value of < 0.05.

Results of two saliva samples were not included in analyses due to the low sample quality. Due to skewed distribution, salivary cytokine concentrations were reported as medians and interquartile ranges. Differences of salivary cytokine concentrations between the obese and normal-weight participants and a pairwise comparison between the groups among different CRS categories were conducted using the Mann–Whitney *U* test. A *p*-value significance level of < 0.05 was used. Multinomial logistic regression was used to determine whether salivary cytokines were associated with obesity, before and after adjusting the model for smoking and periodontal status (CRS). For multinomial logistic regression, cytokine concentrations were converted into tertiles, and the lowest tertile was used as the reference group.

2.5. Ethical Issues

The study was conducted in accordance with the Declaration of Helsinki and approved by the Ethical Committee of the Hospital District of Helsinki and Uusimaa. Written informed consent was obtained from each participant.

3. Results

There was no difference in age, gender, or smoking status between the two study groups, whereas mean BMI was significantly higher in the obese (39.0 kg/m^2) than in the normal-weight (22.9 kg/m^2)

groups ($p < 0.001$) (Table 1). Obese individuals were lower educated ($p = 0.005$) and were more likely to have periodontal disease than their controls ($p = 0.015$).

Table 1. Characteristics of the study groups according to their weight status. Significant differences ($p < 0.05$) are presented in bold.

Demographic and Clinical Parameters	Obese $n = 287$	Normal Weight $n = 293$	p
Age, mean (SD)	55.0 (11.9)	55.5 (12.0)	0.604
Males, n (%)	98 (34.1)	98 (33.4)	0.859
Smokers, n (%)	51 (17.8)	47 (16.0)	0.578
Education level, n (%)			
Low	105 (37.1)	74 (25.3)	**0.005**
Average	94 (33.2)	104 (31.7)	
High	84 (29.7)	115 (39.2)	
BMI, mean (SD)	39.0 (4.1)	22.9 (1.6)	**<0.001**
Periodontitis, n (%)			
Cumulative Risk Score (CRS) I	58 (20.2)	80 (27.3)	**0.015**
Cumulative Risk Score (CRS) II	82 (28.6)	97 (33.1)	
Cumulative Risk Score (CRS) III	147 (51.2)	116 (39.6)	

p-values: Independent samples T-test (age, body mass index (BMI)) and chi-square test (gender, smoking status, educational level, periodontitis).

In the whole population and in smokers, the salivary concentrations of IL-8 were higher (whole population $p = 0.033$; smokers $p = 0.005$) and those of IL-10 were lower (whole population $p = 0.022$; smokers $p = 0.018$) in the obese group than in their controls (Table 2). Other salivary cytokine concentrations did not differ according to weight status. In non-smokers, there was no difference in salivary cytokine concentrations between the groups.

When the study participants were stratified only according to their periodontal status and not by their weight, IL-1Ra and IL-8 concentrations were higher in those with medium or high risk (CRS II and CRS III, $p < 0.001$) of periodontitis, whereas IL-10 and TNF-α concentrations were lower when compared to those with the low risk (CRS I). After weight was taken into account, obese individuals with CRS I had lower IL-10 ($p = 0.043$) and TNF-α ($p = 0.35$) concentrations than their normal-weight controls, while obese individuals with CRS III had higher IL-6 concentrations ($p = 0.011$). Other cytokine concentrations in saliva did not differ between the obese and control groups according to their periodontal status (Table 3).

Table 2. Salivary cytokine concentrations (pg/mL) in the study population and as divided according to smoking status. Significant differences ($p < 0.05$) are presented in bold.

	Whole Population			Smokers			Non-Smokers		
	Obese $n = 285$	Normal Weight $n = 293$	p	Obese $n = 50$	Normal Weight $n = 47$	p	Obese $n = 235$	Normal Weight $n = 246$	p
IL-1Ra	7979 (8712)	7782 (8962)	0.097	7018 (7885)	4877 (4915)	0.036	8566 (9141)	8098 (9136)	0.307
IL-6	3.6 (5.2)	3.3 (4.2)	0.095	3.6 (5.7)	3.6 (6.1)	0.948	3.6 (5.2)	3.2 (4.0)	0.071
IL-8	378 (472)	300 (365)	**0.033**	345 (431)	241 (152)	**0.005**	380 (472)	375 (400)	0.257
IL-10	1.5 (3.0)	2.0 (3.7)	**0.022**	1.7 (3.2)	2.7 (6.5)	**0.018**	1.5 (2.9)	1.9 (3.7)	0.132
TNF-α	10.4 (17.4)	12.6 (18.8)	0.103	10.7 (18.5)	18.3 (23.4)	0.094	10.1 (17.5)	12.4 (17.7)	0.291

All values are given as medians (interquartile ranges). p-values: Mann–Whitney U test.

Table 3. Salivary cytokine concentrations (pg/mL) in the study population divided according to periodontal status. Significant differences ($p < 0.05$) are presented in bold.

	CRS I			CRS II			CRS III		
	Obese $n = 58$	Normal Weight $n = 80$	p	Obese $n = 82$	Normal Weight $n = 97$	p	Obese $n = 147$	Normal Weight $n = 116$	p
IL-1Ra	4419 (2829)	3727 (3497)	0.064	6582 (5478)[a.]	7224 (5402)[a]	0.666	12136 (9387)[a,b]	13045 (10240)[a,b]	0.212
IL-6	3.6 (4.3)	4.5 (4.7)	0.341	2.9 (3.3)	3.0 (3.0)[a]	0.993	4.8 (6.8)[a,b]	3.0 (5.5)	**0.011**
IL-8	169 (127)	168 (125)	0.440	274 (292)[a]	284 (242)[a]	0.682	573 (443)[a,b]	566 (464)[a,b]	0.784
IL-10	3.5 (5.8)	5.7 (8.1)	**0.043**	1.5 (2.8)[a]	2.0 (3.0)[a]	0.078	1.3 (2.2)[a]	1.2 (1.9)[a,b]	0.698
TNF-α	14.4 (23.9)	26.4 (26.4)	**0.035**	9.8 (14.5)[a]	12.4 (13.9)[a]	0.460	8.9 (15.8)[a,b]	10.3 (10.9)[a]	0.841

All values are given as medians (interquartile ranges). In each CRS group, cytokine concentrations were compared between obese and normal-weight groups (p-values). Superscript letters indicate significant differences between the CRS groups in obese and normal-weight individuals as follows: a) A difference in CRS I and b) a difference in CRS II. P-values and superscripts: Mann–Whitney U test.

The multinomial regression model revealed a significant association between obesity and IL-10 concentrations, but the significance was lost after the model was adjusted for smoking and periodontal status (Table 4).

Table 4. Associations of salivary IL-1Ra, IL-6, IL-8, IL-10, and TNF-α tertiles with obesity, before and after adjusting the model for smoking and periodontal status (CRS). Significant associations ($p < 0.05$) are presented in bold.

	Middle Tertile		Highest Tertile	
	Unadjusted	Adjusted	Unadjusted	Adjusted
IL-1Ra	1.5 (1.0–2.3), **0.033**	1.3 (0.9–2.1), 0.194	1.5 (0.9–2.2), 0.06	1.1 (0.7–1.8), 0.722
IL-6	1.3 (0.9–1.9), 0.222	1.3 (0.8–1.9), 0.247	1.2 (0.8–1.8), 0.334	1.2 (0.8–1.8), 0.359
IL-8	1.1 (0.7–1.6), 0.760	0.9 (0.5–1.3), 0.514	1.4 (0.9–2.1), 0.114	0.9 (0.6–1.6), 0.852
IL-10	0.8 (0.5–1.2), 0.264	0.8 (0.5–1.2), 0.287	0.7 (0.4–0.9), **0.042**	0.8 (0.5–1.2), 0.247
TNF-α	0.8 (0.5–1.2), 0.263	0.8 (0.5–1.2), 0.306	0.7 (0.5–1.1), 0.114	0.8 (0.5–1.2), 0.327

Odds ratios (95% confidence intervals) and p-values: Multinomial logistic regression model.

4. Discussion

The main finding of the present study was that, despite periodontal status being worse in obese individuals (BMI of $\geq 35 kg/m^2$) compared to normal-weight controls (BMI of 18.5–25 kg/m^2), the association was not consistently reflected in salivary cytokine concentrations. Instead, the concentrations were merely affected by periodontal status rather than obesity. To our knowledge, this was the first study to investigate potential associations of salivary cytokines with obesity by taking periodontal and smoking states into account.

The relatively large sample size, including 287 severely obese and 293 normal-weight individuals, allowed us to make reliable comparisons of cytokine concentrations in saliva between these groups. However, the cross-sectional study design does not provide any information about the causality between periodontitis, obesity, and cytokines. In addition, the relatively large age range of the study population may have displayed an underestimated effect, since the immune response undergoes remodeling with age. To define the presence of periodontal disease, a novel salivary diagnostic tool, CRS, was used [17]. Its capability has been validated in independent populations twice, showing that the CRS index is more strongly associated with moderate to severe periodontitis than any of the salivary biomarkers alone [21,22]. Finally, as part of the sample collection protocol of this survey study, stimulated saliva samples were collected. The protein concentration was higher in the unstimulated saliva samples than the stimulated saliva samples, however, the unstimulated saliva samples possessed greater inter- and intraindividual variation than the stimulated saliva samples [23].

According to the present study, obese individuals expressed enhanced IL-8 and IL-1Ra but reduced IL-10 concentrations in saliva when compared to normal-weight individuals. This finding was observed especially in smokers. Studies dealing with salivary cytokines in relation to weight are sparse. In a recent small-scale study ($n = 44$), TNF-α concentrations in saliva were shown to be significantly higher in obese than non-obese adults [24]. In obese and non-obese children, on the other hand, salivary TNF-α concentrations did not differ [25]. As both obesity and periodontitis are inflammatory states, it was proposed that obesity-related inflammation could predispose obese subjects to periodontal tissue destruction [12,26]. In the present study, obese individuals displayed mainly CRS II and III, indicating worsened periodontal conditions, more frequently than their normal-weight controls. Nevertheless, there were no consistent differences in the salivary cytokine concentrations between the groups.

In periodontitis, cytokines are mainly released from periodontal tissues after pathogenic bacterial recognition [13,14]. There is also some evidence that adipose tissue-derived cytokines act in a paracrine more than an endocrine manner, and hence do not contribute to cytokine concentrations in the oral cavity [27,28]. It is therefore possible that the local infection of the periodontium has such a strong effect on salivary cytokine concentrations that it overpowers the systemic influence of obesity in statistical analyses. Still, obesity may reinforce the inflammatory response to periodontal pathogens in the periodontium, resulting in an increased susceptibility to periodontitis. It is also possible that the link between obesity and periodontitis is not explained by inflammatory factors.

Obesity and periodontitis share other risk factors, including low socioeconomic status [29]. In the present study, obese individuals were less educated than their controls. This is in line with studies linking educational status to health behaviors as well as eating habits to the prevalence of periodontal disease [29–31]. Obesity-related comorbidities, for example, diabetes mellitus, which is a well-known risk factor for periodontitis [26], could also explain the association between obesity and periodontitis. In our study, diabetic patients were excluded, but the obese individuals may still have insulin resistance, a prediabetic state, which is also a proposed risk factor for periodontitis [32].

In addition to obesity, an unhealthy diet causing weight gain plays a role in the obesity-related inflammatory burden [33–35]. In an experimental rodent model, it was shown that obese rats fed a high-fat and high-carbohydrate diet mimicking the Western diet (known as the "cafeteria diet") caused significantly more advanced alveolar bone loss when compared to non-obese counterparts [34]. In another rodent model, it was observed that a diet enriched with saturated fat was associated with higher inflammatory potential and tissue destruction when compared to a diet high in unsaturated fat in obese mice [34]. Therefore, in future studies regarding obesity and periodontitis in humans, it would be of interest to include the dietary composition of obesity in the analyses.

5. Conclusions

In conclusion, although obese individuals may be prone to have periodontal disease, obesity does not lead to altered cytokine concentrations in saliva. The associations between obesity and salivary cytokine concentrations may be explained by periodontal status and smoking.

Author Contributions: Conceptualization, S.S., U.K.G., and V.S.; data curation, M.G., P.P., A.J., V.S. and P.J.; formal analysis, S.S., U.K.G., M.P., and A.J.; funding acquisition, P.P. and V.S.; methodology, M.G., P.P., M.P., P.J., and E.K.; project administration, U.K.G. and E.K.; resources, V.S. and E.K.; supervision, U.K.G. and E.K.; visualization, S.S.; writing—original draft, S.S. and U.K.G.; writing—review and editing, M.G., P.P., M.P., A.J., V.S., P.J., and E.K.

Funding: Funding for FINRISK and DILGOM Studies was provided by the National Public Health Institute/KTL (currently National Institute for Health and Welfare/THL) through budgetary funds from the government and a grant from the Academy of Finland. DILGOM Study also received funding from the Finnish Dental Society Apollonia and from the State Research Funding. V.S. was supported by the Finnish Foundation for Cardiovascular Research. PP received funding from the Finnish Dental Society Apollonia.

Conflicts of Interest: V.S. participated in a conference trip sponsored by Novo Nordisk and received a honorarium for participating in an advisory board meeting. He also has an ongoing research collaboration with Bayer Ltd (unrelated to the present study). Other authors declare no conflict of interest.

References

1. NCD Risk Factor Collaboration (NCD-RisC). Trends in adult body-mass index in 200 countries from 1975 to 2014: A pooled analysis of 1698 population-based measurement studies with 19.2 million participants. *Lancet* **2016**, *387*, 1377–1396. [CrossRef]
2. Weisberg, S.P.; McCann, D.; Desai, M.; Rosenbaum, M.; Leibel, R.L.; Ferrante, A.W., Jr. Obesity is associated with macrophage accumulation in adipose tissue. *J. Clin. Invest.* **2003**, *112*, 1796–1808. [CrossRef] [PubMed]
3. Ouchi, N.; Parker, J.L.; Lugus, J.J.; Walsh, K. Adipokines in inflammation and metabolic disease. *Nat. Rev. Immunol.* **2011**, *11*, 85–97. [CrossRef] [PubMed]
4. McArdle, M.A.; Finucane, O.M.; Connaughton, R.M.; McMorrow, A.M.; Roche, H.M. Mechanisms of obesity-induced inflammation and insulin resistance: Insights into the emerging role of nutritional strategies. *Front. Endocrinol.* **2013**, *10*, 52. [CrossRef] [PubMed]
5. Schmidt, F.; Weschenfelder, J.; Sander, C.; Minkwitz, J.; Thormann, J.; Chittka, T.; Mergl, R.; Kirkby, K.; Faßhauer, M.; Stumvoll, M.; et al. Inflammatory cytokines in general and central obesity and modulating effects of physical activity. *PLoS ONE* **2015**, *10*, e0121971. [CrossRef]

6. Azizian, M.; Mahdipour, E.; Mirhafez, S.R.; Shoeibi, S.; Nematy, M.; Esmaily, H.; Ferns, G.; Ghayour-Mobarhan, M. Cytokine profiles in overweight and obese subjects and normal weight individuals matched for age and gender. *Ann. Clin. Biochem.* **2016**, *53*, 663–668. [CrossRef]
7. Chae, J.S.; Paik, J.K.; Kang, R.; Kim, M.; Choi, Y.; Lee, S.H.; Lee, J.H. Mild weight loss reduces inflammatory cytokines, leukocyte count, and oxidative stress in overweight and moderately obese participants treated for 3 years with dietary modification. *Nutr. Res.* **2013**, *33*, 195–203. [CrossRef]
8. Chaffee, B.; Weston, S. Association between chronic periodontal disease and obesity: A systematic review and meta-analysis. *J. Periodontol.* **2010**, *81*, 1708–1724. [CrossRef]
9. Suvan, J.; Petrie, A.; Nibali, L.; Darbar, U.; Rakmanee, T.; Donos, N.; D'Aiuto, F. Association between overweight/obesity and increased risk of periodontitis. *J. Clin. Periodontol.* **2015**, *42*, 733–739. [CrossRef]
10. Keller, A.; Rohde, J.; Raymond, K.; Heitmann, B.L. Association between periodontal disease and overweight and obesity. A systematic review. *J. Periodontol.* **2015**, *86*, 766–776. [CrossRef]
11. Nascimento, G.G.; Leite, F.R.; Do, L.G.; Peres, K.G.; Correa, M.B.; Demarco, F.F.; Peres, M.A. Is weight gain associated with the incidence of periodontitis? A systematic review and meta-analysis. *J. Clin. Periodontol.* **2015**, *42*, 495–505. [CrossRef] [PubMed]
12. Falagas, M.; Kompoti, M. Obesity and infection. *Lancet Infect. Dis.* **2006**, *6*, 438–446. [CrossRef]
13. Van Dyke, T.E.; van Winkelhoff, A.J. Infection and inflammation mechanisms. *J. Clin. Periodontol.* **2013**, *40*, S1–S7. [CrossRef] [PubMed]
14. Könönen, E.; Gursoy, M.; Gursoy, U.K. Periodontitis: A Multifaceted Disease of Tooth-Supporting Tissues. *J. Clin. Med.* **2019**, *31*, E1135. [CrossRef]
15. Preshaw, P.M.; Taylor, J.J. How has research into cytokine interactions and their role in driving immune responses impacted our understanding of periodontitis? *J. Clin. Periodontol.* **2011**, *38* (Suppl 11), 60–84. [CrossRef]
16. Kinney, J.; Morelli, T.; Braun, T.; Ramseier, C.; Herr, A.; Sugai, J.; Shelburne, C.; Rayburn, L.; Singh, A.; Giannobile, W. Saliva/pathogen biomarker signatures and periodontal disease progression. *J. Dent. Res.* **2011**, *90*, 752–758. [CrossRef]
17. Gürsoy, U.K.; Könönen, E.; Pussinen, P.; Tervahartiala, T.; Hyvärinen, K.; Suominen, A.; Uitto, V.-J.; Paju, S.; Sorsa, T. Use of host- and bacteria-derived salivary markers in detection of periodontitis: A cumulative approach. *Dis. Markers* **2011**, *30*, 299–306. [CrossRef]
18. Borodulin, K.; Tolonen, H.; Jousilahti, P.; Jula, A.; Juolevi, A.; Koskinen, S.; Kuulasmaa, K.; Laatikainen, T.; Männistö, S.; Peltonen, M.; et al. Cohort profile: The National FINRISK study. *Int. J. Epidemiol.* **2017**, *47*, 696. [CrossRef]
19. Konttinen, H.; Llewellyn, C.; Silventoinen, K.; Joensuu, A.; Männistö, S.; Salomaa, V.; Jousilahti, P.; Kaprio, J.; Perola, M.; Haukkala, A. Genetic predisposition to obesity, restrained eating and changes in body weight: A population-based prospective study. *Int. J. Obes.* **2018**, *42*, 858–865. [CrossRef]
20. Hyvärinen, K.; Laitinen, S.; Paju, S.; Hakala, A.; Suominen-Taipale, L.; Skurnik, M.; Könönen, E.; Pussinen, P. Detection and quantification of five major periodontal pathogens by single copy gene-based real-time PCR. *Innate Immun.* **2009**, *15*, 195–204. [CrossRef]
21. Salminen, A.; Gursoy, U.K.; Paju, S.; Hyvärinen, K.; Mäntylä, P.; Buhlin, K.; Könönen, E.; Nieminen, M.S.; Sorsa, T.; Sinisalo, J. Salivary biomarkers of bacterial burden, inflammatory response, and tissue destruction in periodontitis. *J. Clin. Periodontol.* **2014**, *41*, 442–450. [CrossRef] [PubMed]
22. Gürsoy, U.K.; Pussinen, P.; Salomaa, V.; Syrjäläinen, S.; Könönen, E. Cumulative use of salivary markers with an adaptive design improves detection of periodontal disease over fixed biomarker thresholds. *Acta Odontol. Scand.* **2018**, *76*, 493–496. [CrossRef] [PubMed]
23. Jasim, H.; Olausson, P.; Hedenberg-Magnusson, B.; Ernberg, M.; Ghafouri, B. The proteomic profile of whole and glandular saliva in healthy pain-free subjects. *Sci. Rep.* **2016**, *15*, 39073. [CrossRef] [PubMed]
24. Lehmann-Kalata, A.; Miechowicz, I.; Korybalska, K.; Swora-Cwynar, E.; Czepulis, N.; Łuczak, J.; Orzechowska, Z.; Grzymisławski, M.; Surdacka, A.; Witowski, J. Salivary fingerprint of simple obesity. *Cytokine* **2018**, *110*, 174–180. [CrossRef]
25. Doğusal, G.; Afacan, B.; Bozkurt, E.; Sönmez, I. Gingival crevicular fluid and salivary resistin and tumor necrosis factor-alpha levels in obese children with gingivitis. *J. Periodontol.* **2018**, *89*, 973–982. [CrossRef]
26. Genco, R.; Borgnakke, W. Risk factors for periodontal disease. *Periodontol. 2000* **2013**, *62*, 59–94. [CrossRef]

27. Kern, P.A.; Ranganathan, S.; Li, C.; Wood, L.; Ranganathan, G. Adipose tissue tumor necrosis factor and interleukin-6 expression in human obesity and insulin resistance. *Am. J. Physiol-Endoc. M.* **2001**, *280*, E745–E751. [CrossRef]
28. Wang, P.; Mariman, E.; Renes, J.; Keijer, J. The secretory function of adipocytes in the physiology of white adipose tissue. *J. Cell. Physiol.* **2008**, *216*, 3–13. [CrossRef]
29. Thomson, W.M.; Sheiham, A.; Spencer, A. Sociobehavioral aspects of periodontal disease. *Periodontol. 2000* **2012**, *60*, 54–63. [CrossRef]
30. Laaksonen, M.; Prättälä, R.; Lahelma, E. Sociodemographic determinants of multiple unhealthy behaviours. *Scand. J. Public Healt.* **2003**, *31*, 37–43. [CrossRef]
31. Rezayatmand, R.; Pavlova, M.; Groot, W. Socio-economic aspects of health-related behaviors and their dynamics: A case study for the Netherlands. *Int. J. Health Policy Manag.* **2015**, *5*, 237–251. [CrossRef] [PubMed]
32. Andriankaja, O.; Muñoz-Torres, F.; Vivaldi-Oliver, J.; Leroux, B.; Campos, M.; Joshipura, K.; Pérez, C. Insulin resistance predicts the risk of gingival/periodontal inflammation. *J. Periodontol.* **2018**, *89*, 549–557. [CrossRef] [PubMed]
33. Li, Y.; Lu, Z.; Zhang, X.; Yu, H.; Kirkwood, K.L.; Lopes-Virella, M.F.; Huang, Y. Metabolic syndrome exacerbates inflammation and bone loss in periodontitis. *J. Dent. Res.* **2015**, *94*, 362–370. [CrossRef] [PubMed]
34. Cavagni, J.; de Macedo, I.C.; Gaio, E.J.; Souza, A.; de Molon, R.S.; Cirelli, J.A.; Hoefel, A.L.; Kucharski, L.C.; Torres, I.L.; Rösing, C.K. Obesity and hyperlipidemia modulate alveolar bone loss in wistar rats. *J. Periodontol.* **2016**, *87*, e9–e17. [CrossRef] [PubMed]
35. Muluke, M.; Gold, T.; Kiefhaber, K.; Al-Sahli, A.; Celenti, R.; Jiang, H.; Cremers, S.; Van Dyke, T.; Schulze-Späte, U. Diet-induced obesity and its differential impact on periodontal bone loss. *J. Dent. Res.* **2016**, *95*, 223–229. [CrossRef] [PubMed]

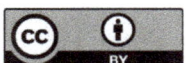

© 2019 by the authors. Licensee MDPI, Basel, Switzerland. This article is an open access article distributed under the terms and conditions of the Creative Commons Attribution (CC BY) license (http://creativecommons.org/licenses/by/4.0/).

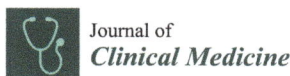 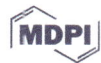

Article

Monitoring of Bactericidal Effects of Silver Nanoparticles Based on Protein Signatures and VOC Emissions from *Escherichia coli* and Selected Salivary Bacteria

Fernanda Monedeiro [1,2,3,†], Paweł Pomastowski [1,2,†], Maciej Milanowski [1,2], Tomasz Ligor [1,2] and Bogusław Buszewski [1,2,*]

1. Department of Environmental Chemistry and Bioanalytics, Faculty of Chemistry, Nicolaus Copernicus University, 87-100 Toruń, Poland; fernandamonedeiro@usp.br (F.M.); pawel_pomastowski@wp.pl (P.P.); milanowski.maciej@gmail.com (M.M.); msd2501@chem.uni.torun.pl (T.L.)
2. Interdisciplinary Centre of Modern Technologies, Nicolaus Copernicus University, 87-100 Toruń, Poland
3. Department of Chemistry, Faculty of Philosophy, Science and Letters of Ribeirão Preto, University of São Paulo, Ribeirão Preto CEP 14040-901, Brazil
* Correspondence: bbusz@chem.uni.torun.pl; Tel.: +48-56-6114308
† Those authors contributed equally to this work.

Received: 13 November 2019; Accepted: 19 November 2019; Published: 19 November 2019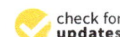

Abstract: *Escherichia coli* and salivary *Klebsiella oxytoca* and *Staphylococcus saccharolyticus* were subjected to different concentrations of silver nanoparticles (AgNPs), namely: 12.5, 50, and 100 µg mL^{-1}. Matrix-assisted laser desorption/ionization–time-of-flight mass spectrometry (MALDI-TOF MS) spectra were acquired after specified periods: 0, 1, 4, and 12 h. For study of volatile metabolites, headspace solid-phase microextraction coupled to gas chromatography/mass spectrometry (HS-SPME-GC-MS) was employed—AgNPs were added to bacteria cultures and the headspace was analyzed immediately and after 12 h of incubation. Principal components analysis provided discrimination between clusters of protein profiles belonging to different strains. Canonical correlation, network analysis, and multiple linear regression approach revealed that dimethyl disulfide, dimethyl trisulfide, 2-heptanone, and dodecanal (related to the metabolism of sulfur-containing amino acids and fatty acids synthesis) are exemplary molecular indicators, whose response variation deeply correlated to the interaction with bacteria. Therefore, such species can serve as biomarkers of the agent's effectiveness. The present investigation pointed out that the used approaches can be useful in the monitoring of response to therapeutic treatment based on AgNPs. Furthermore, biochemical mechanisms enrolled in the bactericidal action of nanoparticles can be applied in the development of new agents with enhanced properties.

Keywords: bacteria; HS-SPME-GC-MS; MALDI-TOF MS; silver nanoparticles; VOCs

1. Introduction

Silver nanoparticles (AgNPs) are widely used in a growing number of industrial and medical applications, such as electronics, food industry, paints, clothing, cosmetics, and medical devices [1,2]. They are well-known antimicrobial agents and their antimicrobial activity against bacteria is attributed to their high reactivity with proteins and initiation of structural changes in the cell wall and membrane. Silver nanoparticles can interact with SH-groups of amino acids and hence inhibit protein synthesis and function. Also, uptake of free silver ions followed by disruption of ATP production and DNA replication is one possible mechanism of toxicity. As a consequence, it leads to inhibition of vital functions and cell death [3,4]. Possible mechanisms of function of silver nanoparticles are described in many publications, however, there are still gaps in the understanding of this phenomenon [4]. Effectiveness of function of AgNPs was investigated by means of various techniques including well and disc diffusion methods and flow cytometry [5–9]. In the current study, we employed matrix-assisted laser desorption/ionization–time-of-flight mass spectrometry (MALDI-TOF MS), which has emerged as a powerful technique for identification of microorganisms [10,11] and for investigation of, for instance, bacterial drug resistance [12]. Protein profiles obtained within the mass range of 2000 to 20,000 Da using MALDI-TOF MS can reflect many physiological states of bacteria [10]. Ag nanoparticles have a dual function in MALDI-TOF MS analyzes, they can serve as a MALDI matrix for enhanced detection of bacteria or as a bactericidal agent. A critical limiting threshold concentration, which governs whether AgNPs would function as an affinity probe or would express bactericidal property, was investigated in the study of Gopal et al. (2011) [13]. Authors conducted their studies using two model bacterial strains: *Escherichia coli* and *Serratia marcescens*. They stated that critical concentration of affinity probes (CCAP) for silver nanoparticles was 1 mL L^{-1} in the case of *E. coli* and 0.5 mL L^{-1} for *S. marcescens*. Above these concentrations, AgNPs became bactericidal for tested bacteria.

Saliva is a biological matrix with promising applications in clinical settings. Its rapid, non-invasive, and cost-effective collection, easy storage and transportation are advantages over other specimens [14,15]. Like serum, saliva contains hormones, antibodies, growth factors, enzymes, microbes, and their products. Consequently, saliva can be considered as a "mirror" of the body for diagnostic purposes of (inter alia) oral diseases [16]. Volatile organic compounds (VOCs) are one of salivary constituents that can indicate various oral conditions, such as halitosis, periodontal disease, lung cancer, and celiac disease [17]. Gas chromatography–mass spectrometry (GC-MS) is a technique which allows detection of VOCs from different niches, including breath, tissues, saliva, or bacteria [18–23]. Solid phase microextraction (SPME) in headspace (HS) variant is a commonly used method for extraction and enrichment of VOCs from many biological matrices [24–26]. Also, VOCs from bacterial strains were analyzed using gas chromatography–mass spectrometry technique. For example, the effect of applied growth medium on emission of volatiles from *E. coli* was investigated in the work of Ratiu et al. (2017) [27]. *Streptococcus pneumoniae* and *Haemophilus influenzae* cultures were identified to find characteristic volatile biomarkers of these bacteria associated with community-acquired pneumonia (CAP) [28]. *Staphylococcus aureus* and *Pseudomonas aeruginosa* were investigated by Filipiak et al. (2012) [29] to find volatile organic compounds from bacteria most frequently found in ventilator-associated pneumonia (VAP) patients. Headspace samples from bacteria were collected and preconcentrated on multibed sorption tubes and analyzed by GC-MS. Once the investigation of bacterial profiles of molecular species can be related with the presence of a specific strain and its metabolic behavior, the features regarding the activity of bactericidal agents can be measured and thoroughly investigated employing the comprehensive evaluation of these profiles.

The aim of the present work is to provide correlated relationships between expressed proteins and volatile metabolites, as a form to assess bactericidal agent performance. Moreover, such knowledge can contribute for elucidation of action mechanism of silver nanoparticles and how they can influence the physiological state of selected bacteria. Growth curves of *E. coli*, *Klebsiella oxytoca*, and *Staphylococcus saccharolyticus* were prepared, then, MALDI-TOF MS technique was employed to obtain proteins profiles of these bacteria and to investigate the addition of selected levels of AgNPs on them. Furthermore, in order to assess alterations in the produced bacterial volatile metabolites, VOCs were investigated by means of HS-SPME-GC-MS, for strains in the unstressed form and after their treatment with silver nanoparticles.

2. Experimental Section

2.1. Instruments

The ultrafleXtreme MALDI-TOF/TOF mass spectrometer (Bruker Daltonik, Bremen, Germany) equipped with a modified Nd:YAG laser (Smartbeam IITM) operating at the wavelength of 355 nm and the frequency of 2 kHz was used to acquire spectra from strains of bacteria by means of two methods and to investigate the interactions between silver nanoparticles and bacterial cells. Optical density (OD) measurements were performed with a DEN-1B Densitometer (Biosan, Riga, Latvia). VITEK® 2 Compact system (bioMérieux, Marcy l'Etoile, France) was employed for identification of salivary bacteria. The GC-MS analyses were carried out using an Agilent 6890A gas chromatograph coupled to an Agilent 5975 Inert XL MSD mass spectrometer (both from Agilent Technologies, Santa Clara, CA, USA). The system was equipped with a Rtx®-5MS w/Integra Guard 30 m × 0.25 mm × 0.25 µm column (Restek Corporation, Bellefonte, PA, USA). Extractions of volatile organic compounds were performed using 65 µm polydimethylsiloxane (PDMS)/divinylbenzene (DVB) fiber (Supelco, Bellefonte, PA, USA). Incubating Microplate Shaker (VWR International, Radnor, PA, USA) was used for incubation of headspace vials with bacterial content.

2.2. Materials

Water LC-MS Chromasolv, ethanol, acetonitrile (ACN), trifluoroacetic acid (TFA), formic acid, and isopropanol were purchased from Sigma Aldrich (Steinheim, Germany). Ultra-pure water from a Milli-Q water system (Millipore, Bedford, MS, USA) was used throughout the work.

All chemicals for MALDI-MS analyses were supplied at the highest commercially available purity from Fluka Feinchemikalien GmbH (part of Sigma Aldrich). Polished steel targets (Bruker Daltonik) were used for sample deposition. α-cyano-4-hydroxycinnamic acid (HCCA; Sigma Aldrich) was employed as a matrix for MALDI analyses (dried droplet method). Bruker bacterial test standard (BTS) was used for external calibration (Bruker Daltonik).

Then, 15 mL sterile polypropylene tubes (ISOLAB, Wertheim, Germany) were used for collection of oral fluid. For identification of salivary bacteria strains, we used 0.45% saline and VITEK® 2 Compact ID Cards for Gram-negative (GN), Gram-positive (GP), and anaerobe corynbacteria (ANC) (bioMérieux). Headspace screw top 20 mL clear vials and magnetic polytetrafluoroethylene (PTFE)/Sil screw caps for headspace vials, 18 mm thread, were purchased from Agilent Technologies.

Three media were used for bacteria cultivation: tryptic soy broth (TSB; Soybean-Casein Digest Medium; Bacto, Sydney, Australia), Mueller Hinton (MH) broth, and M9 (both from Sigma Aldrich). Glucose used as an additive to the minimal medium M9 was purchased from Avantor Performance Materials (Gliwice, Poland). Detailed information regarding media technical aspects can be found elsewhere [30].

The silver nanoparticles used in this study were synthesized in our laboratory and physicochemical characterized previously by Railean-Plugaru et al. (2016) [31]. They were synthesized by the biological method. In comparison with the chemically synthesized one, it was found to be naturally coated with organic deposit, therefore, considered as a biocolloid. The biologically synthesized nanocomposites were tested against 7 different bacterial strains and the antimicrobial activity was found to be dependent on the silver nanocomposite concentrations [9,31].

Two bacterial strains used during investigations, namely: *Escherichia coli* ATCC 25922 and salivary *Klebsiella oxytoca* ATCC 13182 were obtained from POL-AURA (Dywity, Poland). The strain of *Staphylococcus saccharolyticus* was isolated from the saliva of a healthy human oral cavity and identified using VITEK® 2 Compact system, as described by Buszewski et al. (2017) [32].

2.3. Growth Curves of Bacteria

In order to draw the growth curves of the three bacteria, the OD of samples was measured using DEN-1B Densitometer, which provided results in the unit of McFarland (McF). First, three test tubes were filled with 4.8 mL of M9 medium and sterilized by autoclaving. Once the test tubes cooled down, 0.2 mL of prefiltered 10% (m/v) solution of glucose, which served as a source of carbon for bacteria, was added to each tube—the concentration of glucose in the obtained 5 mL of solution was 0.4% (m/v). The content of all test tubes was vortexed for 30 s and the OD of obtained blanks was measured using DEN-1B Densitometer. Then, three loopfuls of bacterial cells were suspended in 1 mL of saline solution to prepare inoculum. Bacterial suspension was thoroughly vortexed for 30 s and the test tubes were inoculated under sterile conditions using 100 µL of the obtained inoculum. Immediately after inoculation, OD at t_0 was determined. Subsequent measurements were performed at t_2, t_4, t_6, t_8, t_{23}, t_{25}, t_{27}, t_{29}, and t_{31}, corresponding to 2, 4, 6, 8, 23, 25, 27, 29, and 31 h of incubation at 37 °C. Growth profiles were assessed for selection of cultivation times to be used in further assays. Such cultivation periods were aimed to refer to the stationary phase of these bacteria, because in this stage the ratio alive/dead is rather constant, thus, the changes observed in the molecular profiles could be ascribed to a metabolic response to the added stressing agent, minimizing the contribution of metabolic alterations due to the growth process.

2.4. MALDI-TOF MS Analysis

MALDI-TOF MS spectra were recorded manually in linear positive mode within m/z range of 3000–30000 and applying the acceleration voltage of 25 kV. All mass spectra were acquired and processed with the dedicated software: flexControl and flexAnalysis, respectively (both from Bruker). Two following experiments with MALDI MS technique were conducted in triplicate during the study.

2.4.1. Comparison of Sample Preparation Methods

The first experiment concerned a comparison between two sample preparation protocols for microorganism profiling, according to the instructions of mass spectrometer manufacturer. The "DIRECT" procedure consists in direct smearing of a sample onto a MALDI target, whereas "EXTRACTION" involves extraction of proteins from a sample with ethanol and formic acid. The HCCA matrix (10 mg mL^{-1}) was prepared in a standard solvent (50% acetonitrile, 47.5% water, 2.5% trifluoroacetic acid). The "DIRECT" procedure was as follows: (i) direct smearing of a small amount of biological material (barely visible) using pipette tips onto a sample spot of a polished steel target, (ii) overlaying the biological material with 1 µL of HCCA matrix solution, (iii) allowing the sample spot to air dry before analysis. The above-mentioned biological material was a precentrifuged (13,000 rpm/RCF = 15,871× g for 2 min) bacterial pellet obtained from 1.5 mL of a liquid culture. For our purpose, we applied three different media (5 mL of TSB, MH, or M9) which were inoculated using a loopful with three bacterial strains and incubated at 37 °C for 24 h. Moreover, we performed OD measurements of a medium alone, a sample after inoculation, and a sample after incubation (next day in the morning). In addition, three types of media alone (TSB, MH, and M9) served as blanks. The "EXTRACTION" protocol was used in the following way: (i) 300 µL of water was transferred into an eppendorf tube containing the biological material and mixed; (ii) then 900 µL of 100% ethanol was added to the tube and mixed thoroughly; (iii) this was followed with centrifugation at 13,000 rpm/RCF = 15,871× g for 2 min and decanting the supernatant; (iv) centrifugation was continued for further 2 min and residual ethanol was removed from the pellet using a pipet; (v) subsequently, 5 µL of 70% formic acid was added to the pellet and mixed thoroughly by pipetting and by vortexing; (vi) 5 µL of acetonitrile was added to the tube and mixed carefully; (vii) the whole was centrifuged at 13,000 rpm/RCF = 15,871× g for 2 min and 1 µL of the supernatant was spotted onto a polished steel target; (viii) the sample was covered with 1 µL of HCCA matrix solution as soon as the sample spot had dried out; (ix) finally, the sample spot was allowed to air dry before analysis. The biological material for "EXTRACTION" method was a precentrifuged (13,000 rpm/RCF = 15,871× g for 2 min) bacterial pellet obtained from 1.5 mL of a liquid culture with MH medium. In this part of the experiment we used only MH medium (5 mL) inoculated using a loopful with three bacteria and incubated at 37 °C for 24 h. The samples were smeared onto a MALDI target in triplicate. Extract from pure MH was used as a blank in this step.

2.4.2. Influence of AgNPs on MALDI-TOF MS Profiles of the Selected Bacteria

A total of 150 mL of MH medium was prepared and shared between three Erlenmeyer flasks (50 mL in each). After sterilization, each portion of medium was inoculated with two loopfuls of bacterial cells (approximately 1×10^6 of cells) of *E. coli*, *K. oxytoca*, and *S. saccharolyticus* individual strains and placed into a shaker at 37 °C for 8, 15, or 18 h, depending on strain type (based on growth curves experiments). Then, under sterile conditions, nine sterilized test tubes received 10 mL of liquid culture each. Immediately, silver nanoparticles were added and vortexed to obtain the final silver concentration of 12.5, 50, and 100 µg mL^{-1}. After that, OD measurements were performed. Next, all test tubes with their content were placed into an incubator at 37 °C for a specified period of time, namely: 0, 1, 4, and 12 h, then 1.5 mL of each solution was transferred to an Eppendorf tube and centrifuged at 13,000 rpm/RCF = 15,871× g for 2 min. The supernatant was removed and the bacterial pellet was subjected to the "EXTRACTION" technique (treatment of a sample using ethanol and formic acid).

2.5. Gas Chromatography–Mass Spectrometry (GC-MS)

A total of 4 mL of sterilized MH broth was inoculated with 100 µL of a bacterial suspension (already cultured bacteria, under 37 °C for 8, 15, or 18 h, depending on strain type) of *E. coli*, *K. oxytoca*, and *S. saccharolyticus* in the medium (100 µL of pure medium was used as a blank). Before application of AgNPs, OD of the inoculum was always measured and was approximately 1.5 McF. Immediately, silver nanoparticles were added to obtain the final concentration of 12.5 and 50 µg mL^{-1}. All four headspace vials (three with bacteria and one with a blank) were placed into an incubator at 37 °C with continuous shaking. Then, the vials were taken out immediately (t = 0) and after 12 h (t = 12). VOCs were extracted at 37 °C for 45 min, using 65 µm PDMS/DVB fiber. All GC-MS experiments were done in triplicate. Helium with a flow rate of 1.1 mL min^{-1} was the carrier gas and temperature of the split–splitless injector was set at 240 °C. The oven temperature program was as follows: The initial temperature of 40 °C was kept for 3 min, then ramped at 10 °C min^{-1} to 300 °C and kept at this last temperature for 5 min. Spectra acquisition was performed within m/z range of 30–300 with electron ionization (EI) at 70 eV; both the ion source and the transfer line temperature was set at 250 °C.

2.6. Data Processing and Statistical Analysis

Part of the data processing and statistical analysis was performed in R environment, using RStudio v.1.1.463 console. GC-MS raw data (CDF format) was processed using the "xcms" package, peaks were detected in the shift region of 10 ppm, applying the "centWave" method. As result, a database displaying retention time and corresponding area for extracted ion chromatogram (EIC) was obtained. Peaks arising from medium blanks in different incubation times were subtracted from the related bacterial samples. Peak identification was performed using NIST11, for each peak detected belonging to the same retention time—a match factor of at least 750/1000 was considered. From MALDI-TOF MS data, the 100 most intense and corresponding signals were annotated and ion database was created manually.

A comparison between MALDI-TOF MS raw spectra (mzXML format) obtained from bacterial extract before and after AgNPs addition was performed by calculation of the spectrum similarity score (SSS), with usage of "OrgMassSpecR" package in default mode. Heatmaps based on the area of ions, associated with hierarchical cluster analysis using the Spearman method, were built employing "gplots" package.

Canonical correlation analysis (CCA) is a multivariate ordination analysis used to provide sample correlations between two sets of variables. This method was employed to relate the variation in the fold-change of VOCs and proteins ions after the treatment with nanoparticles. The analysis was conducted using representative features ($p < 0.05$, indicated by Mann–Whitney test), "vegan" package was applied to run CCA function.

Network analysis was performed using "igraph" package, in order to provide visualization of the connections between both sets of data. Spearman's coefficients were used to produce the edges between nodes representing protein ions and VOCs, which presented statistically relevant ($p < 0.05$) change in their response after the addition of nanoparticles.

With the usage of IBM SPSS Statistics v.24, Spearman correlation coefficient was calculated between triplicates to verify the reproducibility of the obtained profiles. Principal components analysis (PCA) was carried out to assess the distribution of MALDI-TOF MS profiles according to strain. Mann–Whitney U test was performed to indicate discriminating features. Linear regression was used to create a model able to predict the extension of AgNPs interaction with bacteria. Detailed information regarding used R packages and input formats, as well as employed databases are available in Supplementary Materials.

3. Results

3.1. Determination of Growth Curves

Figure S1 depicts growth curves of three selected bacteria grown in minimal medium M9 with glucose as a source of carbon. Based on the assessed curves, further experiments were conducted using 8, 15, or 18 h of cultivation of E. coli, K. oxytoca, and S. saccharolyticus, respectively. Bacteria at the given times were at the beginning of the stationary phase. Previous experiments reported growth profiles of the selected bacteria using MH medium [33–35].

3.2. Comparison of Procedures: Direct Smearing Versus Extraction and Medium Selection

Straight and clear baseline with negligible signals recorded in the acquired spectra were seen for all tested growth media (M9, MH, and TSB) after using "DIRECT" and "EXTRACTION" (MH only) protocols (Figure S2). Figure S3 demonstrates an exemplary comparison of MALDI-TOF MS spectra of *E. coli* cultured in M9, MH, and TSB media, obtained using "DIRECT" method. The presented observations for *E. coli* are typical for our selected bacterial strains. M9 was found to be the most effective medium among the used growth media. The number of peaks reached almost 100. Moreover, the number of signals with signal-to-noise ratio (S/N) greater than or equal to 10 was 77. Only 33 and 34 signals with such defined S/N were recorded for MH and TSB medium, respectively. However, for further MALDI-TOF MS investigations concerning addition of silver nanoparticles, we selected MH medium, since it provided the best results in the simultaneously conducted GC-MS study (Figure 1).

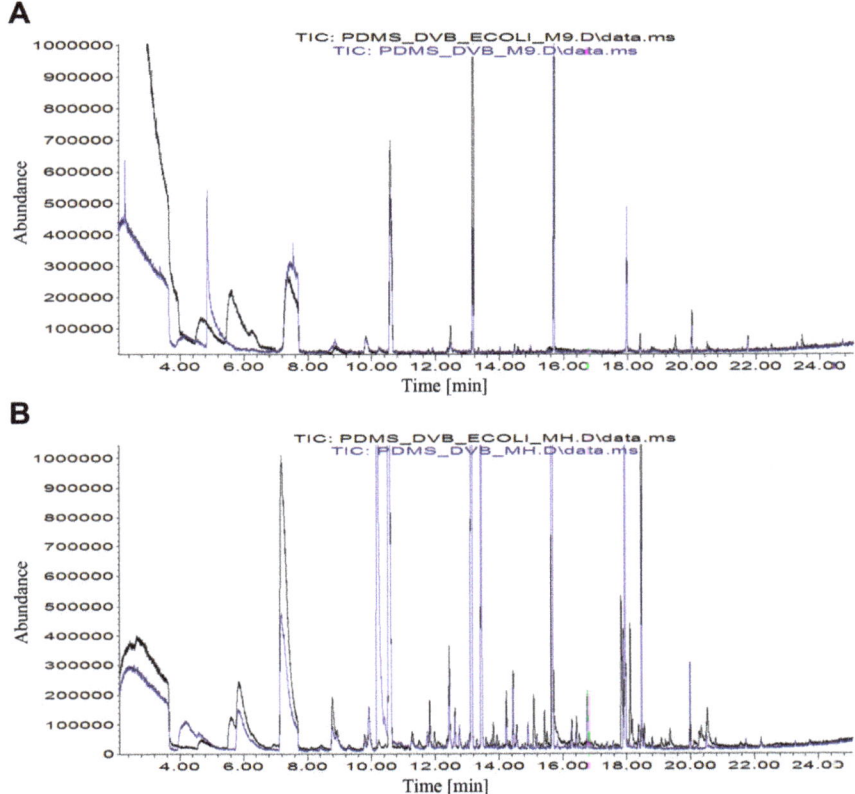

Figure 1. Comparison of overlaid gas chromatography–mass spectrometry (GC-MS) chromatograms obtained for (**A**) *E.coli* bacterium + M9 medium (black) versus pure M9 medium (blue) and (**B**) *E.coli* bacterium + Mueller Hinton (MH) medium (black) versus pure MH medium (blue).

Figure 2 shows a comparison between the two applied sample preparation techniques with the example of E. coli.

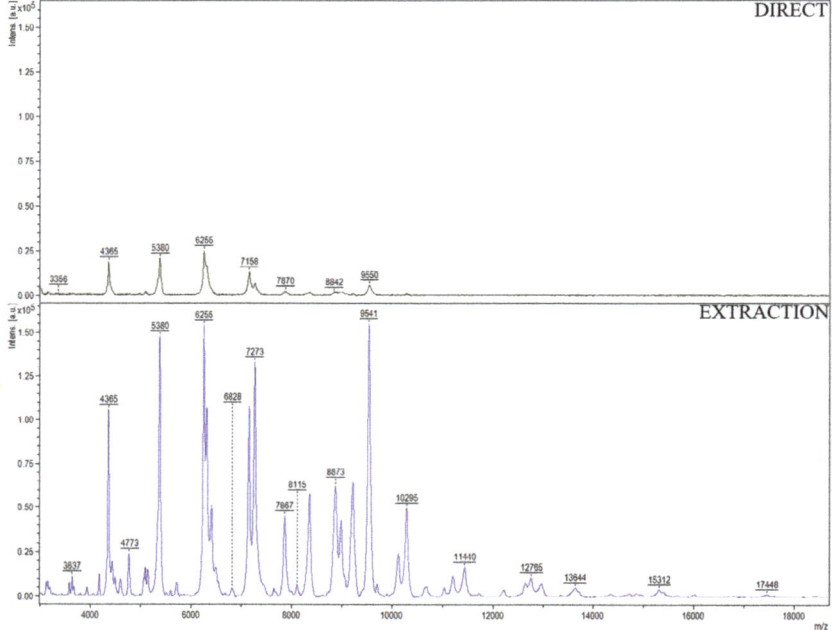

Figure 2. Representative (from triplicate experiment) matrix-assisted laser desorption/ionization–time-of-flight mass spectrometry (MALDI-TOF MS) spectra of *E. coli* in MH medium obtained using the "DIRECT" and "EXTRACTION" procedure.

The differences between MALDI-TOF MS spectra include both the number of detected peaks and their intensity. For E. coli, in the "EXTRACTION" method, we recorded 54 signals with S/N greater than or equal 10. On contrary, for the "DIRECT" procedure, we found only 33 peaks fulfilling this requirement. Moreover, signals obtained for the "EXTRACTION" procedure were several times more intense than the values for the "DIRECT" technique. Similar observations were extended to the other studied bacteria. It indicates that sample treatment using ethanol and formic acid is far more efficient than the method consisting in direct smearing of a sample onto a MALDI target.

3.3. Influence of Silver Nanoparticles on MALDI-TOF MS Spectra and HS-SPME-GC-MS Chromatograms of the Selected Bacteria

To investigate the influence of AgNPs on MALDI-TOF MS spectra of the three model bacteria, the following tests were conducted. In this part of the study, the "EXTRACTION" technique was applied for sample preparation of each bacterial strain, as it was found to be superior to the "DIRECT" procedure in the previous experiment.

Regarding MALDI-TOF MS experiments, the prepared database displayed 1928 most relevant ions, ranging from 3013 to 17,449 *m/z*. In GC-MS data, ions addressed as belonging to medium, GC column material, or fiber coating were subtracted from the database, resulting in a total number of 281 computed ions, ranging from 32 to 298 *m/z*.

Figure 3 presents the PCA score plot obtained for different protein ions profiles acquired under the mentioned experimental conditions, for each bacterial strain. Profiles belonging to an individual bacterial strain were clearly separated from others, highlighting the discriminative power of ribosomal profiles in bacteria identity. However, still being possible to observe that the performed assays were capable of significantly altering such profiles, in this case, the distinction between the 3 strains was explained by only 14% of the variance.

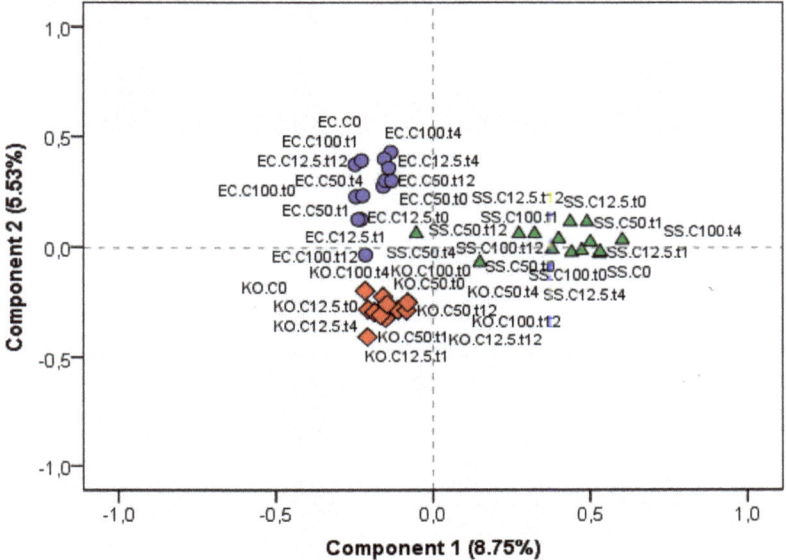

Figure 3. Principal component analysis (PCA) plot of protein ions profiles acquired by MALDI-TOF MS experiments, where diamonds, triangles, and circles represent *K. oxytoca* (KO), *S. saccharolyticus* (SS), and *E. coli* (EC), respectively.

Heatmaps referring to protein ions profiles (Figure 4A) and VOC profiles (Figure 4B) allow inspection of the distribution of ions detected in each experiment. Hierarchical cluster analysis evidencing the similarity between these individual profiles and segregation according to bacterial strain were observed in data extracted both by MALDI-TOF MS and GC-MS results. The ions constituting the profiles were grouped in clusters, which correspond to the main distribution behaviors identified along the samples.

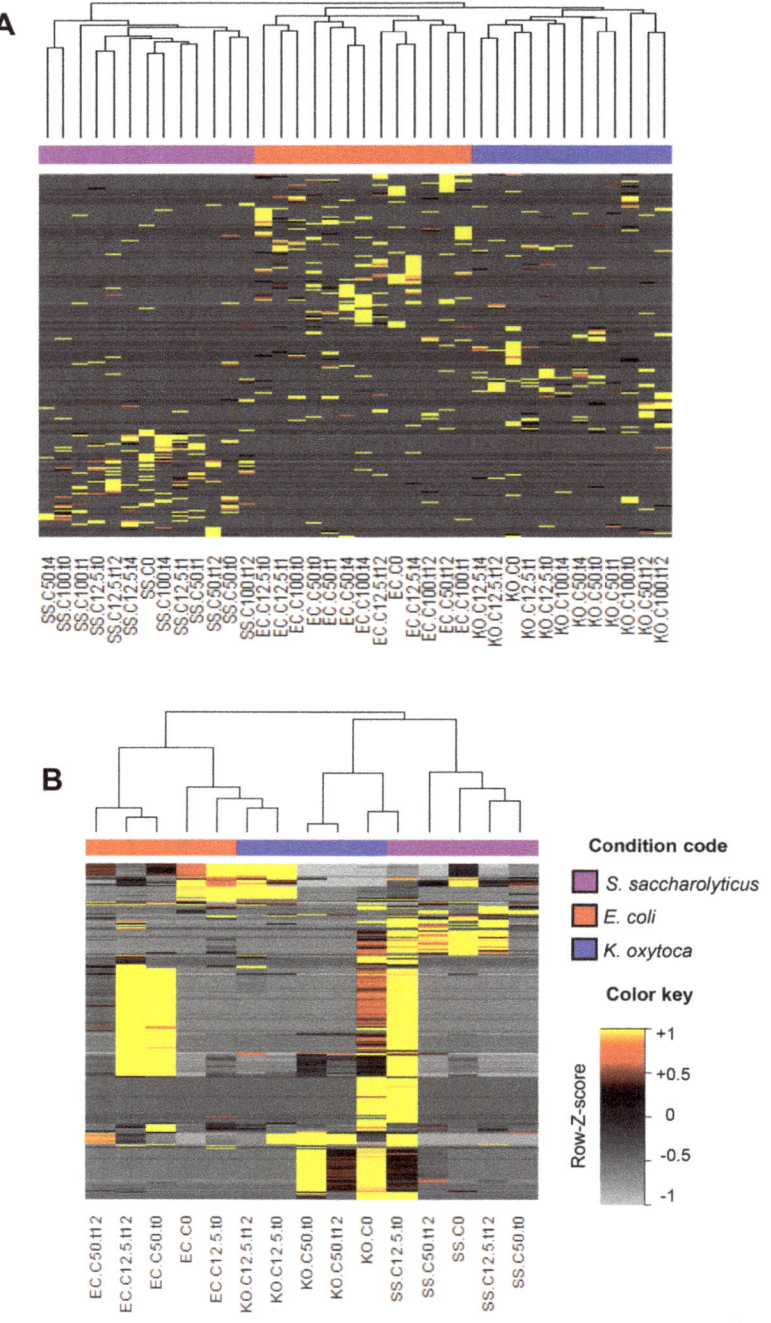

Figure 4. Heatmaps and hierarchical cluster analysis of protein ions (**A**) and volatile organic compound (VOC) profiles (**B**), based on ion areas extracted from MALDI-TOF MS spectra and GC-MS chromatograms, respectively; Horizontal axis = conducted assays, using different bacterial strains, vertical axis = ions organized in clusters.

In order to objectively quantify the overall changes in MALDI-TOF MS spectra after the addition of nanoparticles, the SSS parameter was assessed. The average SSSs calculated for each experiment are displayed in Figure 5. This parameter mathematically represents the average level of similarity between spectra acquired for unstressed strain and the same strain after supplementation with AgNPs. The clusters on the right side of the matrix are based on Euclidian distance and represent more similar behaviors during assay with nanoparticles.

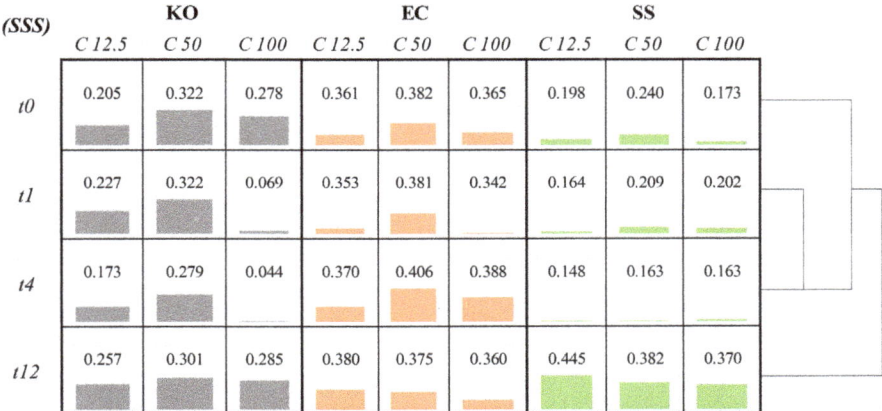

Figure 5. Matrix presenting average values of spectra similarity score (SSS), concerning comparison between unstressed spectrum and assays using silver nanoparticles (AgNPs) at 12.5, 50, and 100 μg mL^{-1}, for periods of time 0, 1, 4, and 12 h. Gray, orange, and green bars refer to *K. oxytoca* (KO), *S. saccharolyticus* (SS), and *E. coli* (EC), respectively; C—concentration (μg mL^{-1}); t—time (h).

For *K. oxytoca*, it can be seen that for concentration 100 μg mL^{-1}, the biggest changes in profiles were obtained for 1 and 4 h after supplementation with AgNPs. After 12 h, an adaptation to the stressing agent is observable resulting in an increased spectrum similarity score to the original native strain. For lower concentrations (12.5 and 50 μg mL^{-1}), *K. oxytoca* manifested stronger resistance to applied silver nanoparticles. *E. coli* was the most resistant for concentration 50 μg mL^{-1}, bigger alternations were noticed for the remaining concentrations. On the other hand, *S. saccharolyticus* appeared to be the most susceptible to added AgNPs. This strain reacted the most in the first hours after supplementation of silver nanoparticles. The strain showed tolerance to stressing agent only after 12 h of influence, regardless of the used concentration. In a general view, the apex of interaction of AgNPs with intercellular portion can be addressed as the higher studied concentration (100 μg mL^{-1}), associated to the incubation time of 4 h for *K. oxytoca* and *S. saccharolyticus* and 1 h for *E. coli*. Once 12 h of incubation was reached, an overall tendency to return to the untreated-like profile is observed for all strains.

With the aim to investigate how the alterations produced in profiles of bacterial proteins are reflected in the VOCs distribution, canonical correlation analysis (CCA) and direct correlation analysis using the Pearson method were conducted. The results are showed in Figure 6. The CCA plot (Figure 6A), along its CCA1 and CCA2 axes, was able to explain 37.71% of the variance of a matrix combining MALDI-TOF MS and GC-MS data. This observation points out the possible relation between VOCs emitted by bacteria and their pattern of small proteins. Although it can be understood that this fraction of proteins is not the only factor governing VOCs production, some particular ions seemed to be closely related to the detected volatiles, regardless of the studied strain. In this plot, length and angle of arrows are related to the contribution of a certain variable to the axes. Variables not accompanied by arrows displayed much weaker influence score than others, not being depicted in the automatically scaled graph. The compounds that presented to be the most affected by bacterial ribosomes were dimethyl disulfide, 2-heptanone, 2-undecanol, dimethyl trisulfide, 3-methyl-1-butanol, 1-nonanol, and 2-tetradecanol. While dimethyl disulfide, 2-heptanone, and 1-nonanol can be interpreted as having correlated behavior between them in the three studied bacteria, hexanal and 2-tetradecanol, for example, demonstrated a much more diverse trend than the aforementioned compounds. Figure 6B allows a visual inspection of the nature of the main connections between the two classes of variables. Variables not showed in this network are those that did not present strong or relevant correlation and, in contrast to the last approach, only individual interactions were considered. Interdependency relationships can be also examined: according to the network analysis, the compounds 2-heptanone, 3-methyl-1-butanol, 3-methylbutanoic acid, and dodecanal have their levels associated with many different related proteins—from this, it can be concluded that their expression is associated with intricate factors.

With basis on what was demonstrated concerning the strong correlations between emitted VOCs and protein ions, it was assumed that the levels of such VOCs could provide indirect information about effectiveness of interaction of the bactericidal agent and colonizing bacteria. This approach has potential usefulness in the monitoring of therapeutic response to antimicrobial treatment. Multiple linear regression analysis was conducted in order to create a model based on VOCs as biomarkers of the extension of AgNPs interaction with bacteria. Level of interaction was used as criterion, using 100-SSS*100 as parameter, since it is related to the percentage of modification of unstressed bacterial spectra. VOCs' responses common to all strains were employed as predictors. As a result, Equation (1) was obtained, with R (coefficient of correlation between observed and predicted values) = 0.89, adjusted R square = 0.79, and standard error of estimate = ±4.10. Such parameters indicate good precision of the generated model:

$$\% \text{ of agent effectiveness} = 42.9 + 1.6 \times 10^{-5} \times A_{\text{dimethyl disulfide}} \\ - 2.8 \times 10^{-7} \times A_{\text{dimethyl trisulfide}} + 5.3 \times 10^{-6} \times A_{\text{2-heptanone}} - 2.9 \times 10^{-8} \times A_{\text{dodecanal}}. \tag{1}$$

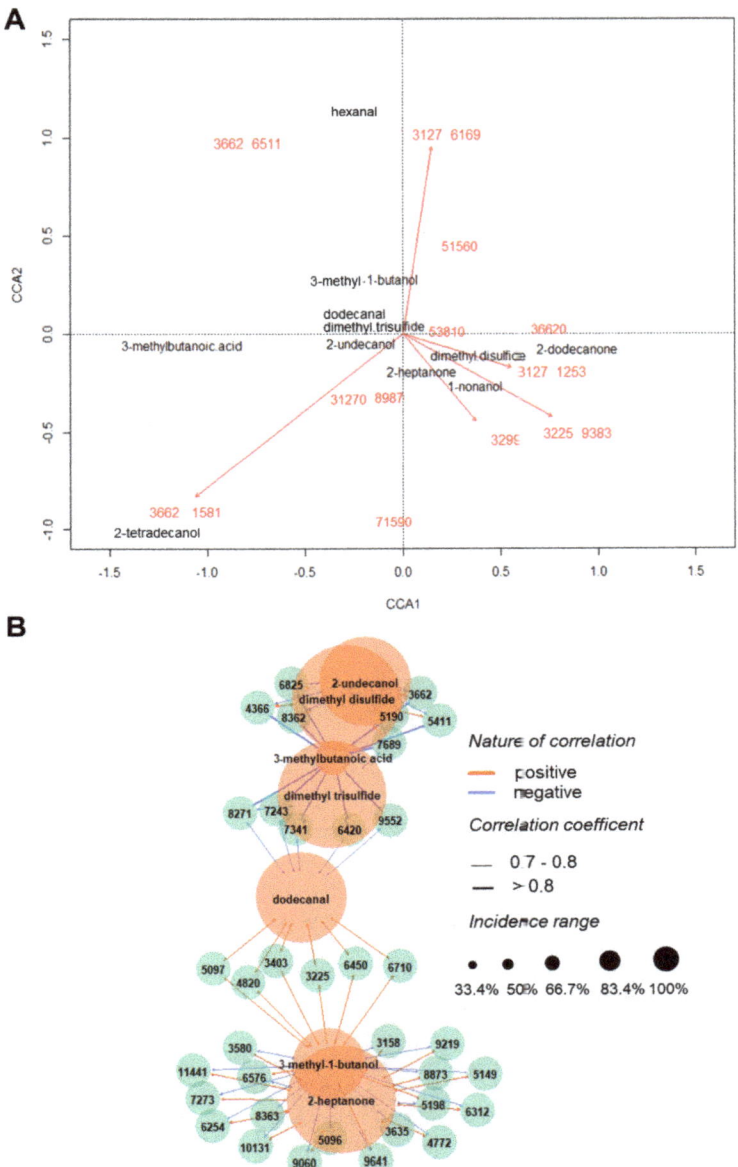

Figure 6. (**A**) Canonical correlation analysis (CCA) biplot showing the correspondence of the main protein ions (red) with emitted VOCs (black), where CCA1 = 22.43% and CCA2 = 15.28%; (**B**) Correlation network depicting main relevant connections (rho ≥ |0.7|) between MALDI-TOF MS ions and identified volatiles.

4. Discussion

The subjects of our work were: *Escherichia coli* (Gram-negative bacterium) and salivary *Klebsiella oxytoca* (Gram-negative bacterium) and *Staphylococcus saccharolyticus* (Gram-positive bacterium). The differences between cell wall structure of Gram-positive and Gram-negative bacteria are essential in the mechanism of interaction of silver nanoparticles with the surface and the inner part of bacteria. Combined effects of AgNPs and antibiotics (ampicillin, kanamycin, erythromycin, and chloramphenicol) were investigated in the Fayaz et al. (2010) study for bactericidal activity against test strains using the disc diffusion method with Mueller Hinton agar plates [36]. In another work, silver colloid nanoparticles synthesized by reduction of $[Ag(NH_3)_2]^+$ complex cation by four saccharides revealed high antimicrobial and bactericidal activity against both Gram-positive and Gram-negative bacteria, including *E. coli* and methicillin-resistant *S. aureus*. Authors claimed that the size of particles and very low concentration of silver are crucial to exhibit bactericidal properties of these nanoparticles [37]. In Krishna et al. (2015), antibacterial activity of silver nanoparticles was tested against the two pathogenic strains *Salmonella typhi* and *Salmonella paratyphi* by well-diffusion method. Complex of AgNPs-ofloxacin demonstrated the augmented effect in comparison to separated components [38]. The example of work showing superiority of Gram-positive bacteria over Gram-negative ones in the meaning of resistance against AgNPs is described by Fayaz et al. (2010).

The tested bacteria from this study were two Gram-positive cocci and two Gram-negative rods, including *E. coli*. The antibacterial activity for all antibiotics (especially ampicillin) increased in the presence of AgNPs against test strains. The minimum inhibitory concentration (MIC) evaluated for synergistic effect of AgNPs and antibiotics showed increased less significant influence on growth of Gram-positive bacteria than on Gram-negative species. Cell wall of Gram-positive bacteria is characterized by a thick peptidoglycan layer (~20–80 nm), whereas in Gram-negative bacteria, the peptidoglycan layer is thinner (~7–8 nm) and sandwiched between two layers of periplasmic space and covered by an outer membrane composed by liposaccharides (LPSs) portion. The Gram-negative wall is considered as more susceptible than the Gram-positive one, because the negative charges liposaccharides are attracted toward the positive relative charge available on silver nanoparticles. Moreover, Fayaz et al. (2010) described also negatively charged AgNPs which can attack this type of bacteria by metal depletion [36]. It was found that *E. coli* cells are more prone to increased permeability after ethylenediaminetetraacetate disodium (EDTA) treatment. Liberation of LPS molecules from outer cell membrane are caused by higher metal depletion which weakens maintaining the assembly of the LPSs in membrane [39]. On the contrary, Gram-positive bacteria with thicker layer of peptidoglycan are more resistant to AgNPs because of hindered penetration of nanoparticles and fewer anchoring points for the AgNPs. The layer is highly composed of rigid structure of linear polysaccharide cross-linked by short peptides [36]. The AgNPs-ampicillin complex prevents unwinding of cellular DNA by preferential binding of silver atoms with cells' DNA [40].

Our work showed that Gram-positive *S. saccharolyticus* was the most resistant strain at all tested AgNPs levels against the remaining Gram-negative ones, when the highest incubation time (12 h) is considered (Figure 5). However, at shorter incubation times *E. coli* and *K. oxytoca* appeared to be more insusceptible for AgNPs influence as reflected in protein profiles acquired by MALDI-TOF MS. After 12 h, bacterial strains exhibited behavior more similar to unstressed ones, deprived of the effect of nanoparticles. Another observation was the fact that both Gram-negative bacteria were more resistant at medium concentration (50 μg mL^{-1}) of AgNPs. Such remark was not noticed for *S. saccharolyticus* strain, making this bacterium more distinctive. In recent work of Al-Sharqi et al. (2019), authors investigated antibacterial efficiencies of photoactivated and not-enhanced AgNPs against *E. coli* and *S. aureus*. Cells not treated with silver nanoparticles served as controls. The results for unmodified *E. coli* show that after 24 h of treatment with 12.5 μg mL^{-1} AgNPs, bacterial growth was observed to be 93.33% ± 2.88%. Along with increasing concentration of AgNPs, the microbial number decreased significantly reaching the lowest value of survival viability in the level of 76% ± 1.73% for 100 μg mL^{-1} [41]. Our work confirms that with long time of incubation, *E. coli* is more susceptible for AgNPs influence with increasing level of added stressing agent, from 12.5 to 100 µg mL^{-1}.

Protein patterns were processed to obtain heatmap and hierarchical cluster analysis (Figure 4A) that allowed to distinguish three separate clusters belonging to each bacterial strain. It proves effectiveness and appropriateness of the conducted research and shows potential applicability in differentiation purposes. Using lysozyme-stabilized silver nanoparticles, Ashraf et al. (2014) were able to differentiate some of the strains (two *Salmonella enterica*, two *Klebsiella pneumoniae*, four *P. aeruginosa*, two *E. coli*) within the same bacterial species based upon the difference of their antimicrobial activity [42].

The bactericidal effect of silver nanoparticles consists in several mechanisms; (1) AgNPs can adhere onto the surface of cell wall, resulting in membrane damage and altered transport activity [43]. Penetration of cell membrane causes the increased permeability and death of the cell [44]. The damage to membranes is the result of the formation of irregular-shaped pits in the cell surface due to release of LPS molecules [39,45]. (2) Anchoring of silver to cell membrane also inhibits cell wall formation [44,46]. (3) AgNPs modulate cellular signal system and induce oxidative stress caused by generation of reactive oxygen species (ROS) and free radicals [46]. These free radicals can increase porosity of the cell membrane, leading to damage and cell death [44]. (4) AgNPs can be the source of silver ions released by themselves. These Ag$^+$ are able to react with thiol groups of enzymes and proteins causing inactivation of them [44,45]. (5) Silver nanoparticles tend to react also with phosphorus-containing compounds such as DNA and prevent its replication as well as cell division and respiratory chain processes [44,45,47]. (6) AgNPs modulate cellular signaling by dephosphorylation of protein substrates in bacteria, resulting in inhibition of cell growth [48]. Finally, changes in nucleoid of bacteria are leading to DNA fragmentation, cell cycle arrest, apoptosis, and inflammatory response [49]. Silver nanoparticles are characterized by many physico-chemical parameters affecting their antimicrobial effectiveness, such as shape, size, concentration, particle dispersion state, and surface charge [43,49].

MALDI-TOF MS technique is often used to identify bacterial strains in timesaving manner and pure culture isolation, such as model organism *E. coli* [50] and other Gram-positive, Gram-negative, anaerobic bacteria and mycobacteria [51,52]. In our work, we applied MALDI-TOF MS technique to obtain protein profiles of bacteria after treatment with silver nanoparticles. In the work of Lok et al. (2006), proteomic analyzes using two-dimensional gel electrophoresis (2-DE) and MS identification revealed that short exposure of *E. coli* cells to AgNPs resulted in alterations in the expressions of a panel of envelope proteins and heat shock proteins (like 30S ribosomal subunit S6) [50]. Twenty protein patterns were identified by MALDI-TOF MS technique from the set of recombinant, human cDNA expression products, together with native proteins isolated from crude mouse brain extracts [53]. Peptide mass fingerprint (PMF) searching of databases appeared to be a cost-effective solution for protein identification purposes. Sixty-two proteins in unsequenced parasitic nematodes were identified by MALDI-TOF MS after evaluation of expressed sequence tag (EST) datasets [54]. This technique was also used, for example, to characterize proteomic patterns in serum from ovarian cancer and healthy control group [55].

MALDI-TOF MS was a suitable technique to investigate binding bare and carbonate-coated AgNPs to the purified tryptophanase (TNase) fragments from *E. coli* to characterize the effect of surface modifications on the binding. It was showed that binding of the protein to AgNPs may sterically block access to the active site caused by lost enzymatic activity of TNase [56]. Using MALDI mass spectra, authors could evaluate the TNase' enhanced affinity for AgNPs, similarly to our present experiments with protein patterns. Metabolic alterations in bacteria after supplementation with nanoparticles were the subject of interest in the study of Gopal et al. (2013) [57]. They examined the interaction of five types of nanoparticles (Ag, NiO, Pt, TiO$_2$, and ZnO) with *P. aeruginosa* and *S. aureus* and postulated two mechanisms of interaction of the above-mentioned NPs with these two pathogenic bacterial strains. The approach consisting in addition of AgNPs at 0 h of bacterial growth, and incubation with bacteria when they grow in the medium, enabled effective interaction of *P. aeruginosa* with unmodified NPs. For *S. aureus*, NPs were added to fully grown bacterial cultures and incubated—a method similar to the one used in our work. In this case, in MALDI-MS spectra, many bacterial peaks were observed. The changes of proteomic profiles were also the object of the researcher interest in the work of He et al. [58]. They carried out the proteomic analysis of graphene-based silver nanoparticles (AgNPs–GE) together with silver nitrate on *P. aeruginosa*. MALDI–TOF/TOF MS was used to identify proteins from bacteria as outcome of 2-DE experiments with silver agents. Authors discovered seven proteins being induced and nine proteins being suppressed by AgNPs–GE.

The effect of the addition of silver nanoparticles on the *S. aureus* strain was again studied in the work of Chudobova et al. (2013) [59]. These researchers conducted a basic characterization of this strain and found out that AgNPs caused considerable inhibition of the growth of *S. aureus*. The authors proposed two methods for determination of silver nanoparticles inhibition effect: using the growth curves and measurements of inhibition zones. Protein fingerprints for the identification of untreated and silver-supplemented *S. aureus* were obtained by MALDI/TOF mass spectra. The usage of the MALDI-TOF MS technique was extended in the more recent work of Chudobova et al. (2015), dedicated to *S. aureus* strain [60]. They focused on examination of the influence of selected heavy metal ions (Ag^+, Cu^{2+}, Cd^{2+}, Zn^{2+}, and Pb^{2+}) at several concentration levels using biochemical methods and mass spectrometry. Additional peaks in silver-fortified bacteria were found in the obtained MALDI-TOF MS spectra demonstrating modifications at the protein level.

The above-mentioned studies are clear examples of how silver ions or nanoparticles may affect the metabolic and proteomic profiles of bacteria, changes in which are visible using the MALDI MS technique. In the present work, a new approach was introduced: MALDI MS and GC-MS data were processed and correlated using statistical methods that allowed to characterize patterns of small proteins and volatile metabolites associated with the interaction of nanoparticles with bacteria.

Once it was demonstrated that VOC profiles are able to reflect metabolic alterations in bacterial cells, the effective changes in the response of detected volatiles were evaluated. Figure 7 shows VOCs presenting statistically relevant ($p < 0.05$) difference in their distribution when varying amounts of AgNPs were added to the bacterial culture. It is reasonable to assume that the consequences of the presence of nanoparticles in the medium can vary depending on the examined microorganism. For example, after AgNPs addition, dimethyl disulfide levels increased for *K. oxytoca*, and decreased for the other two bacteria; for dimethyl trisulfide, the other sulfur containing metabolite, an opposite trend is observed.

Bacterial strain		KO		EC		SS	
Main related pathways	VOC	C 12.5	C 50	C 12.5	C 50	C 12.5	C 50
Pyruvate metabolism, Glycolysis or Gluconeogenesis	acetic acid	pr	pr	ab	ab	ns	ns
Ehrlich pathway (aminoacid metabolism)	3-methylbutanoic acid	−1.1	ab	ns	ns	ns	ns
	3-methyl-1-butanol	+0.8	+1.8	−0.5	−1.1	ab	ab
Metabolism of sulfur containing aminoacids	dimethyl disulfide	+3.8	+4.0	−1.2	−1.2	−1.2	−0.9
	dimethyl trisulfide	−4.1	−0.9	+0.2	+4.2	+2.8	+3.3
Fatty alcohols formation (fatty acids biosynthesis)	1-nonanol	+1.3	+4.0	ns	ns	−1.4	−3.0
Sencodary alcohols formation (fatty acids biosynthesis)	2-undecanol	−4.7	−5.7	+1.0	+1.8	−1.4	ab
	2-tetradecanol	ab	−1.6	ns	ns	ns	ns
Methyl ketones formation (fatty acids biosynthesis)	2-heptanone	−4.1	−3.9	−0.4	+2.0	−4.8	−5.0
	2-octanone	ab	ab	ns	ns	ns	ns
	2-dodecanone	ab	ns	+1.2	−3.1	−5.2	ns
Fatty aldehydes formation (fatty acids biosynthesis), Lipid peroxidation	hexanal	−5.7	ab	−7.1	ab	ns	ns
	dodecanal	+0.5	+4.4	+1.0	ab	ns	+4.4

Figure 7. Combination of charts showing altered VOCs and addressed bacterial metabolic pathways, where numbers inside boxes display the base 2 logarithm of fold-change calculated with respect to the response in untreated strain; pr = produced only after AgNPs addition, ab = absent after AgNPs addition, ns = not significant alteration ($p > 0.05$), KO—*K. oxytoca*, EC—*E. coli*, SS—*S. saccharolyticus*, C—concentration (µg mL^{-1}), VOC—volatile organic compound [61].

The origin of volatiles released by three investigated bacteria is mainly a modification of products of the fatty acid biosynthetic pathway, like hydrocarbons, alcohols, and ketones (Figure 8) [61].

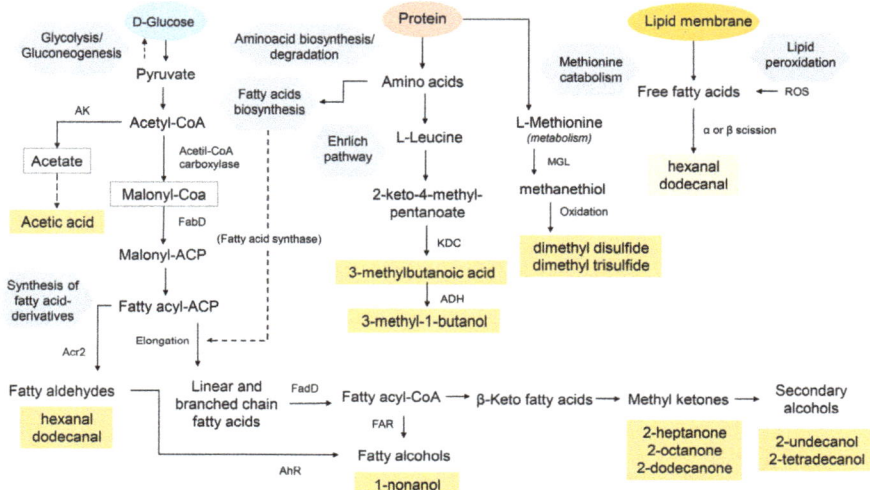

Figure 8. Scheme showing main pathways related to volatile organic metabolites which presented relevant alterations in their responses due to nanoparticles supplementation (AK—acetate kinase; KDC—2-keto acid decarboxylase; ADH—alcohol dehydrogenase; FAR—fatty acid reductase; FabD—malonyl-CoA:ACP transacylase; FadD—fatty acyl-CoA synthase; AhR—aryl hydrocarbon receptor; Acr2—acyl-CoA reductase; MGL—methionine-γ-lyase; ROS—reactive oxygen species).

Volatile organic compounds secreted from *E. coli* were the object of interest of several researchers who used multiple techniques to investigate the headspace of bacteria. Tait et al. (2014) [62] performed optimization of conditions of HS-SPME-GC-MS analysis of *E. coli* VOCs and evaluated the effect of a culture medium type, SPME fiber type, and the employed GC column on the obtained results. Furthermore, volatile profiles of *E. coli* were investigated in the work of Umber et al. (2013) [63] who found elevated levels of such compounds as: dimethyl disulfide, dimethyl trisulfide, and 1-propanol in the headspace of bacteria in LB broth. These volatiles were not observed in chromatograms obtained from *E. coli*/blood mixture. In our research, we detected these three compounds both in the untreated and AgNPs-supplemented strain of *E. coli*.

VOCs from *K. oxytoca* and other species were studied using ion-molecule reaction–mass spectrometry (IMR-MS) by Dolch et al. (2012) [64]. This method allowed to conduct a short analysis time of 3 min per vial and showed the possibility of process automation. For identification of human pathogenic bacteria (like *E. coli* and *K. oxytoca*), Jünger et al. 2012 used multi-capillary column–ion mobility spectrometry (MCC-IMS). Comparisons of volatilomes were confirmed by thermal desorption–gas chromatography–mass spectrometry (TD-GC-MS). VOC patterns from bacteria enabled fast and cost-effective discrimination of investigated pathogens [65]. Another technique employed for volatile extraction from *E. coli*, *K. oxytoca*, and *P. aeruginosa* was a static head-space-sampler (SHS) coupled to a sensory perception system (SPS). Carrillo and Durán 2019 used this method for distinguish polluted water samples after statistical approaches such as pattern recognition techniques [66].

S. saccharolyticus is a bacterial strain responsible for, inter alia, the production of volatile compounds in spoilt mango fruits. GC-MS analyzes revealed the presence of eleven and sixteen volatile organic constituents in healthy and spoilt ripe mango fruits, respectively [67]. There are no other studies concerning volatile profiling of *S. saccharolyticus*. In recent work of Brüggemann et al. (2019),

S. saccharolyticus isolates from blood cultures and prosthetic joint infection specimens were detected and their genomes were sequenced and analyzed. They found that the closest relative of *S. saccharolyticus* is *Staphylococcus capitis* with an average nucleotide identity of 80%. Moreover, *S. saccharolyticus* manifests host tissue-invasive potential and is associated with prosthetic joint infections [68].

5. Conclusions

The reported results confirm that the MALDI-TOF MS technique is an appropriate tool for investigating the influence of silver nanoparticles on metabolism of selected bacterial strains. The comparison between spectra acquired from untreated and silver-enhanced bacteria revealed that addition of AgNPs led to significant changes in their metabolic profiles. Such metabolic alterations were attested by distinguished variations in the emitted bacterial metabolites assessed using GC-MS.

It was demonstrated that interaction between AgNPs and bacteria is deeply associated to the concentration of nanoparticles, incubation time, and strain nature, considerations to be evaluated for the employment of such species as bactericidal agent in medical practice.

Statistical approaches performed in this work reinforced the relation between ribosomal profiles and strain identity, besides that, combination between the variation in protein ion data and VOC patterns allowed the observation of alterations in bacterial inner part closely related with produced volatile metabolites.

Moreover, it can be concluded that the usage of molecular profiles is a promising tool in monitoring of bactericidal performance during infection treatment and to investigate the associated biochemical mechanisms.

Supplementary Materials: The following are available online at http://www.mdpi.com/2077-0383/8/12/2024/s1, Figure S1: Growth curves of three bacteria cultured in M9 medium. Figure S2: MALDI-TOF MS blanks obtained for (A) M9, MH and TSB media using "DIRECT" protocol and for (B) MH medium after "EXTRACTION" method. Figure S3: Representative (from triplicate experiment) MALDI-TOF MS spectra of E. coli in M9, MH and TSB media obtained using "DIRECT" procedure.

Author Contributions: Conceptualization, F.M. and P.P.; Methodology, F.M. and P.P.; Software, F.M. and M.M.; Validation, F.M., P.P. and M.M.; Formal analysis, F.M., P.P. and M.M.; Investigation, F.M. and P.P.; Resources, F.M. and P.P.; Data curation, F.M.; Writing—Original draft preparation, F.M., P.P. and M.M.; Writing—Review and editing, T.L. and B.B.; Visualization, F.M. and M.M.; Supervision, T.L. and B.B.; Project administration, B.B.; Funding acquisition, P.P.

Funding: This work was financially supported by National Science Centre in frame of Opus 14 project No. 2017/27/B/ST4/02628 (2018-2021).

Conflicts of Interest: The authors declare no conflict of interest.

References

1. Ahamed, M.; AlSalhi, M.S.; Siddiqui, M.K.J. Silver nanoparticle applications and human health. *Clin. Chim. Acta* **2010**, *411*, 1841–1848. [CrossRef] [PubMed]
2. León-Silva, S.; Fernández-Luqueño, F.; López-Valdez, F. Silver Nanoparticles (AgNP) in the Environment: A Review of Potential Risks on Human and Environmental Health. *Water Air Soil Pollut.* **2016**, *227*, 306. [CrossRef]
3. Quinteros, M.A.; Cano Aristizábal, V.; Dalmasso, P.R.; Paraje, M.G.; Páez, P.L. Oxidative stress generation of silver nanoparticles in three bacterial genera and its relationship with the antimicrobial activity. *Toxicol. Vitr.* **2016**, *36*, 216–223. [CrossRef] [PubMed]
4. Durán, N.; Durán, M.; de Jesus, M.B.; Seabra, A.B.; Fávaro, W.J.; Nakazato, G. Silver nanoparticles: A new view on mechanistic aspects on antimicrobial activity. *Nanomed. Nanotechnol. Biol. Med.* **2016**, *12*, 789–799. [CrossRef] [PubMed]
5. Saxena, J.; Sharma, P.K.; Sharma, M.M.; Singh, A. Process optimization for green synthesis of silver nanoparticles by Sclerotinia sclerotiorum MTCC 8785 and evaluation of its antibacterial properties. *Springerplus* **2016**, *5*, 861. [CrossRef]

6. Krishnaraj, C.; Ji, B.J.; Harper, S.L.; Yun, S. Il Plant extract-mediated biogenic synthesis of silver, manganese dioxide, silver-doped manganese dioxide nanoparticles and their antibacterial activity against food- and water-borne pathogens. *Bioprocess Biosyst. Eng.* **2016**, *39*, 759–772. [CrossRef]
7. Aazam, E.S.; Zaheer, Z. Growth of Ag-nanoparticles in an aqueous solution and their antimicrobial activities against Gram positive, Gram negative bacterial strains and Candida fungus. *Bioprocess Biosyst. Eng.* **2016**, *39*, 575–584. [CrossRef]
8. Hong, W.; Li, L.; Liang, J.; Wang, J.; Wang, X.; Xu, S.; Wu, L.; Zhao, G.; Xu, A.; Chen, S. Investigating the environmental factors affecting the toxicity of silver nanoparticles in Escherichia coli with dual fluorescence analysis. *Chemosphere* **2016**, *155*, 329–335. [CrossRef]
9. Railean-Plugaru, V.; Pomastowski, P.; Rafinska, K.; Wypij, M.; Kupczyk, W.; Dahm, H.; Jackowski, M.; Buszewski, B. Antimicrobial properties of biosynthesized silver nanoparticles studied by flow cytometry and related techniques. *Electrophoresis* **2016**, *37*, 752–761. [CrossRef]
10. Singhal, N.; Kumar, M.; Kanaujia, P.K.; Virdi, J.S. MALDI-TOF mass spectrometry: An emerging technology for microbial identification and diagnosis. *Front. Microbiol.* **2015**, *6*, 791. [CrossRef]
11. Rahi, P.; Prakash, O.; Shouche, Y.S. Matrix-assisted laser desorption/ionization time-of-flight mass-spectrometry (MALDI-TOF MS) based microbial identifications: Challenges and scopes for microbial ecologists. *Front. Microbiol.* **2016**, *7*, 1359. [CrossRef] [PubMed]
12. Yari, S.; Tasbiti, A.H.; Ghanei, M.; Shokrgozar, M.A.; Vaziri, B.; Mahdian, R.; Yari, F.; Bahrmand, A. Proteomic analysis of sensitive and multi drug resistant Mycobacterium tuberculosis strains. *Microbiology* **2016**, *85*, 350–358. [CrossRef]
13. Gopal, J.; Wu, H.F.; Lee, C.H. The bifunctional role of Ag nanoparticles on bacteria—A MALDI-MS perspective. *Analyst* **2011**, *136*, 5077–5083. [CrossRef] [PubMed]
14. Lima, D.P.; Diniz, D.G.; Moimaz, S.A.S.; Sumida, D.H.; Okamoto, A.C. Saliva: Reflection of the body. *Int. J. Infect. Dis.* **2010**, *14*, 184–188. [CrossRef] [PubMed]
15. Lee, Y.H.; Wong, D.T. Saliva: An emerging biofluid for early detection of diseases. *Am. J. Dent.* **2009**, *22*, 241–248. [PubMed]
16. Chiappin, S.; Antonelli, G.; Gatti, R.; De Palo, E.F. Saliva specimen: A new laboratory tool for diagnostic and basic investigation. *Clin. Chim. Acta* **2007**, *383*, 30–40. [CrossRef]
17. Milanowski, M.; Pomastowski, P.; Ligor, T.; Buszewski, B. Saliva–Volatile Biomarkers and Profiles. *Crit. Rev. Anal. Chem.* **2017**, *47*, 251–266. [CrossRef]
18. Buszewski, B.; Ulanowska, A.; Ligor, T.; Jackowski, M.; Kłodzińska, E.; Szeliga, J. Identification of volatile organic compounds secreted from cancer tissues and bacterial cultures. *J. Chromatogr. B Anal. Technol. Biomed. Life Sci.* **2008**, *868*, 88–94. [CrossRef]
19. Soini, H.A.; Klouckova, I.; Wiesler, D.; Oberzaucher, E.; Grammer, K.; Dixon, S.J.; Xu, Y.; Brereton, R.G.; Penn, D.J.; Novotny, M.V. Analysis of Volatile Organic Compounds in Human Saliva by a Static Sorptive Extraction Method and Gas Chromatography-Mass Spectrometry. *J. Chem. Ecol.* **2010**, *36*, 1035–1042. [CrossRef]
20. Boots, A.W.; Smolinska, A.; van Berkel, J.J.B.N.; Fijten, R.R.R.; Stobberingh, E.E.; Boumans, M.L.L.; Moonen, E.J.; Wouters, E.F.M.; Dallinga, J.W.; Van Schooten, F.J. Identification of microorganisms based on headspace analysis of volatile organic compounds by gas chromatography–mass spectrometry. *J. Breath Res.* **2014**, *8*, 027106. [CrossRef]
21. Neerincx, A.H.; Geurts, B.P.; Van Loon, J.; Tiemes, V.; Jansen, J.J.; Harren, F.J.M.; Kluijtmans, L.A.J.; Merkus, P.J.F.M.; Cristescu, S.M.; Buydens, L.M.C.; et al. Detection of Staphylococcus aureus in cystic fibrosis patients using breath VOC profiles. *J. Breath Res.* **2016**, *10*, 046014. [CrossRef] [PubMed]
22. Amann, A.; Miekisch, W.; Schubert, J.; Buszewski, B.; Ligor, T.; Jezierski, T.; Pleil, J.; Risby, T. Analysis of Exhaled Breath for Disease Detection. *Ann. Rev. Anal. Chem.* **2014**, *7*, 455–482. [CrossRef] [PubMed]
23. Buszewski, B.; Kęsy, M.; Ligor, T.; Amann, A. Human exhaled air analytics: Biomarkers of diseases. *Biomed. Chromatogr.* **2007**, *21*, 553–566. [CrossRef] [PubMed]
24. Kusano, M.; Mendez, E.; Furton, K.G. Development of headspace SPME method for analysis of volatile organic compounds present in human biological specimens. *Anal. Bioanal. Chem.* **2011**, *400*, 1817–1826. [CrossRef]
25. Kusano, M.; Mendez, E.; Furton, K.G. Comparison of the Volatile Organic Compounds from Different Biological Specimens for Profiling Potential. *J. Forensic Sci.* **2013**, *58*, 29–39. [CrossRef]

26. Brown, J.S.; Prada, P.A.; Curran, A.M.; Furton, K.G. Applicability of emanating volatile organic compounds from various forensic specimens for individual differentiation. *Forensic Sci. Int.* **2013**, *226*, 173–182. [CrossRef]
27. Ratiu, I.A.; Ligor, T.; Bocos-Bintintan, V.; Al-Suod, H.; Kowalkowski, T.; Rafińska, K.; Buszewski, B. The effect of growth medium on an Escherichia coli pathway mirrored into GC/MS profiles. *J. Breath Res.* **2017**, *11*, 036012. [CrossRef]
28. Filipiak, W.; Sponring, A.; Baur, M.M.; Ager, C.; Filipiak, A.; Wiesenhofer, H.; Nagl, M.; Troppmair, J.; Amann, A. Characterization of volatile metabolites taken up by or released from Streptococcus pneumoniae and Haemophilus influenzae by using GC-MS. *Microbiol (U.K.)* **2012**, *158*, 3044–3053. [CrossRef]
29. Filipiak, W.; Sponring, A.; Baur, M.; Filipiak, A.; Ager, C.; Wiesenhofer, H.; Nagl, M.; Troppmair, J.; Amann, A. Molecular analysis of volatile metabolites released specifically by staphylococcus aureus and pseudomonas aeruginosa. *BMC Microbiol.* **2012**, *12*, 113. [CrossRef]
30. Jo Zimbro, M.; Power, D.A.; Sharon Miller, M.; Wilson, G.E.; Johnson, J.A. *Difco TM & BBL TM Manual of Microbiological Culture*, 2nd ed.; Becton, Dickinson and Company: Sparks, MD, USA, 2009.
31. Railean-Plugaru, V.; Pomastowski, P.; Wypij, M.; Szultka-Mlynska, M.; Rafinska, K.; Golinska, P.; Dahm, H.; Buszewski, B. Study of silver nanoparticles synthesized by acidophilic strain of Actinobacteria isolated from the of Picea sitchensis forest soil. *J. Appl. Microbiol.* **2016**, *120*, 1250–1263. [CrossRef]
32. Buszewski, B.; Milanowski, M.; Ligor, T.; Pomastowski, P. Investigation of bacterial viability from incubated saliva by application of flow cytometry and hyphenated separation techniques. *Electrophoresis* **2017**, *38*, 2081–2088. [CrossRef] [PubMed]
33. Burian, A.; Erdogan, Z.; Jandrisits, C.; Zeitlinger, M. Impact of pH on Activity of Trimethoprim, Fosfomycin, Amikacin, Colistin and Ertapenem in Human Urine. *Pharmacology* **2012**, *90*, 281–287. [CrossRef] [PubMed]
34. Freney, J.; Kloos, W.E.; Hajek, V.; Webster, J.A.; Bes, M.; Brun, Y.; Vernozy-Rozand, C. Recommended minimal standards for description of new staphylococcal species. *Int. J. Syst. Bacteriol.* **1999**, *49*, 489–502. [CrossRef] [PubMed]
35. Knöppel, A.; Knopp, M.; Albrecht, L.M.; Lundin, E.; Lustig, U.; Näsvall, J.; Andersson, D.I. Genetic adaptation to growth under laboratory conditions in Escherichia coli and Salmonella enterica. *Front. Microbiol.* **2018**, *9*, 756. [CrossRef]
36. Fayaz, A.M.; Balaji, K.; Girilal, M.; Yadav, R.; Kalaichelvan, P.T.; Venketesan, R. Biogenic synthesis of silver nanoparticles and their synergistic effect with antibiotics: A study against gram-positive and gram-negative bacteria. *Nanomed. Nanotechnol. Biol. Med.* **2010**, *6*, 103–109. [CrossRef]
37. Panáček, A.; Kvítek, L.; Prucek, R.; Kolář, M.; Večeřová, R.; Pizúrová, N.; Sharma, V.K.; Nevěčná, T.; Zbořil, R. Silver Colloid Nanoparticles: Synthesis, Characterization, and Their Antibacterial Activity. *J. Phys. Chem. B* **2006**, *110*, 16248–16253. [CrossRef]
38. Krishna, G.; Kumar, S.S.; Pranitha, V.; Alha, M.; Charaya, S. Biogenic synthesis of silver nanoparicles and their synergistic effect with antibiotics: A study against Salmonella SP. *Int. J. Pharm. Pharm. Sci.* **2015**, *7*, 84–88.
39. Amro, N.A.; Kotra, L.P.; Wadu-Mesthrige, K.; Bulychev, A.; Mobashery, S.; Liu, G.Y. High-resolution atomic force microscopy studies of the Escherichia coli outer membrane: Structural basis for permeability. *Langmuir* **2000**, *16*, 2789–2796. [CrossRef]
40. Batarseh, K.I. Anomaly and correlation of killing in the therapeutic properties of siliver (I) chelation with glutamic and tartaric acids. *J. Antimicrob. Chemother.* **2004**, *54*, 546–548. [CrossRef]
41. Al-Sharqi, A.; Apun, K.; Vincent, M.; Kanakaraju, D.; Bilung, L.M. Enhancement of the Antibacterial Efficiency of Silver Nanoparticles against Gram-Positive and Gram-Negative Bacteria Using Blue Laser Light. *Int. J. Photoenergy* **2019**, *2019*, 2528490. [CrossRef]
42. Ashraf, S.; Chatha, M.; Ejaz, W.; Janjua, H.; Hussain, I. Lysozyme-coated silver nanoparticles for differentiating bacterial strains on the basis of antibacterial activity. *Nanoscale Res. Lett.* **2014**, *9*, 565. [CrossRef] [PubMed]
43. Dakal, T.C.; Kumar, A.; Majumdar, R.S.; Yadav, V. Mechanistic basis of antimicrobial actions of silver nanoparticles. *Front. Microbiol.* **2016**, *7*, 1831. [CrossRef] [PubMed]
44. Prabhu, S.; Poulose, E.K. Silver nanoparticles: Mechanism of antimicrobial action, synthesis, medical applications, and toxicity effects. *Int. Nano Lett.* **2012**, *2*, 32. [CrossRef]
45. Sondi, I.; Salopek-Sondi, B. Silver nanoparticles as antimicrobial agent: A case study on E. coli as a model for Gram-negative bacteria. *J. Colloid Interface Sci.* **2004**, *275*, 177–182. [CrossRef]

46. Gumel, A.M.; Surayya, M.M.; Yaro, M.N.; Waziri, I.Z.; Amina, A.A. Biogenic synthesis of silver nanoparticles and its synergistic antimicrobial potency: An overview. *J. Appl. Biotechnol. Bioeng.* **2019**, *6*, 22–28.
47. Morones, J.R.; Elechiguerra, J.L.; Camacho, A.; Holt, K.; Kouri, J.B.; Ramírez, J.T.; Yacaman, M.J. The bactericidal effect of silver nanoparticles. *Nanotechnology* **2005**, *16*, 2346–2353. [CrossRef]
48. Shrivastava, S.; Bera, T.; Roy, A.; Singh, G.; Ramachandrarao, P.; Dash, D. Characterization of enhanced antibacterial effects of novel silver nanoparticles. *Nanotechnology* **2007**, *18*, 225103. [CrossRef]
49. Liao, C.; Li, Y.; Tjong, S. Bactericidal and Cytotoxic Properties of Silver Nanoparticles. *Int. J. Mol. Sci.* **2019**, *20*, 449. [CrossRef]
50. Lok, C.N.; Ho, C.M.; Chen, R.; He, Q.Y.; Yu, W.Y.; Sun, H.; Tam, P.K.H.; Chiu, J.F.; Che, C.M. Proteomic analysis of the mode of antibacterial action of silver nanoparticles. *J. Proteome Res.* **2006**, *5*, 916–924. [CrossRef]
51. Siller-Ruiz, M.; Hernández-Egido, S.; Sánchez-Juanes, F.; González-Buitrago, J.M.; Muñoz-Bellido, J.L. Fast methods of fungal and bacterial identification. MALDI-TOF mass spectrometry, chromogenic media. *Enferm. Infecc. Microbiol. Clin. (Engl. Ed.)* **2017**, *35*, 303–313. [CrossRef]
52. Yang, Y.; Lin, Y.; Qiao, L. Direct MALDI-TOF MS Identification of Bacterial Mixtures. *Anal. Chem.* **2018**, *90*, 10400–10408. [CrossRef] [PubMed]
53. Egelhofer, V.; Büssow, K.; Luebbert, C.; Lehrach, H.; Nordhoff, E. Improvements in protein identification by MALDI-TOF-MS peptide mapping. *Anal. Chem.* **2000**, *72*, 2741–2750. [CrossRef] [PubMed]
54. Millares, P.; LaCourse, E.J.; Perally, S.; Ward, D.A.; Prescott, M.C.; Hodgkinson, J.E.; Brophy, P.M.; Rees, H.H. Proteomic profiling and protein identification by MALDI-TOF mass spectrometry in unsequenced parasitic nematodes. *PLoS ONE* **2012**, *7*, e33590. [CrossRef] [PubMed]
55. Swiatly, A.; Horala, A.; Hajduk, J.; Matysiak, J.; Nowak-Markwitz, E.; Kokot, Z.J. MALDI-TOF-MS analysis in discovery and identification of serum proteomic patterns of ovarian cancer. *BMC Cancer* **2017**, *17*, 1–9. [CrossRef] [PubMed]
56. Wigginton, N.S.; De Titta, A.; Piccapietra, F.; Dobias, J.A.N.; Nesatyy, V.J.; Suter, M.J.F.; Bernier-Latmani, R. Binding of silver nanoparticles to bacterial proteins depends on surface modifications and inhibits enzymatic activity. *Environ. Sci. Technol.* **2010**, *44*, 2163–2168. [CrossRef] [PubMed]
57. Gopal, J.; Manikandan, M.; Hasan, N.; Lee, C.-H.; Wu, H.-F. A comparative study on the mode of interaction of different nanoparticles during MALDI-MS of bacterial cells. *J. Mass Spectrom.* **2013**, *48*, 119–127. [CrossRef]
58. He, T.; Liu, H.; Zhou, Y.; Yang, J.; Cheng, X.; Shi, H. Antibacterial effect and proteomic analysis of graphene-based silver nanoparticles on a pathogenic bacterium Pseudomonas aeruginosa. *BioMetals* **2014**, *27*, 673–682. [CrossRef]
59. Chudobova, D.; Maskova, D.; Nejdl, L.; Kopel, P.; Rodrigo, M.A.M.; Adam, V.; Kizek, R. The effect of silver ions and silver nanoparticles on Staphylococcus aureus. *Microb. Pathog. Strateg. Combat. Sci. Technol. Educ.* **2013**, *1*, 728–735.
60. Chudobova, D.; Dostalova, S.; Ruttkay-Nedecky, B.; Guran, R.; Rodrigo, M.A.M.; Tmejova, K.; Krizkova, S.; Zitka, O.; Adam, V.; Kizek, R. The effect of metal ions on Staphylococcus aureus revealed by biochemical and mass spectrometric analyses. *Microbiol. Res.* **2015**, *170*, 147–156. [CrossRef]
61. Schulz, S.; Dickschat, J.S. Bacterial volatiles: The smell of small organisms. *Nat. Prod. Rep.* **2007**, *24*, 814–842. [CrossRef]
62. Tait, E.; Perry, J.D.; Stanforth, S.P.; Dean, J.R. Identification of volatile organic compounds produced by bacteria using HS-SPME-GC-MS. *J. Chromatogr. Sci.* **2014**, *52*, 363–373. [CrossRef] [PubMed]
63. Umber, B.J.; Shin, H.-W.; Meinardi, S.; Leu, S.-Y.; Zaldivar, F.; Cooper, D.M.; Blake, D.R. Gas signatures from Escherichia coli and Escherichia coli-inoculated human whole blood. *Clin. Transl. Med.* **2013**, *2*, 13. [CrossRef] [PubMed]
64. Dolch, M.E.; Hornuss, C.; Klocke, C.; Praun, S.; Villinger, J.; Denzer, W.; Schelling, G.; Schubert, S. Volatile compound profiling for the identification of Gram-negative bacteria by ion-molecule reaction-mass spectrometry. *J. Appl. Microbiol.* **2012**, *113*, 1097–1105. [CrossRef] [PubMed]
65. Jünger, M.; Vautz, W.; Kuhns, M.; Hofmann, L.; Ulbricht, S.; Baumbach, J.I.; Quintel, M.; Perl, T. Ion mobility spectrometry for microbial volatile organic compounds: A new identification tool for human pathogenic bacteria. *Appl. Microbiol. Biotechnol.* **2012**, *93*, 2603–2614. [CrossRef] [PubMed]
66. Carrillo, J.; Durán, C. Fast identification of bacteria for quality control of drinking water through a static headspace sampler coupled to a sensory perception system. *Biosensors* **2019**, *9*, 23. [CrossRef] [PubMed]

67. Ibrahim, A.D.; Oyeleke, B.S.; Muhammad, U.K.; Aliero, A.; Yakubu, S.E.; Safiyanu, H.M. Microorganisms Associated with Volatile Organic Compound Production in Spoilt Mango Fruits. *Indones. J. Biotechnol.* **2011**, *16*, 11–16.
68. Brüggemann, H.; Poehlein, A.; Brzuszkiewicz, E.; Scavenius, C.; Enghild, J.J.; Al-Zeer, M.A.; Brinkmann, V.; Jensen, A.; Söderquist, B. Staphylococcus saccharolyticus Isolated from Blood Cultures and Prosthetic Joint Infections Exhibits Excessive Genome Decay. *Front. Microbiol.* **2019**, *10*, 478. [CrossRef]

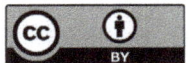

© 2019 by the authors. Licensee MDPI, Basel, Switzerland. This article is an open access article distributed under the terms and conditions of the Creative Commons Attribution (CC BY) license (http://creativecommons.org/licenses/by/4.0/).

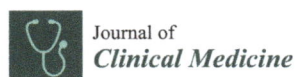

Article

Salivary IL-6 mRNA is a Robust Biomarker in Oral Squamous Cell Carcinoma

Ildikó Judit Márton [1,*], József Horváth [2], Péter Lábiscsák [2], Bernadett Márkus [2], Balázs Dezső [3], Adrienn Szabó [4], Ildikó Tar [5], József Piffkó [6], Petra Jakus [6], József Barabás [7], Péter Barabás [7], Lajos Olasz [8], Zsanett Kövér [8], József Tőzsér [2], János Sándor [9], Éva Csősz [2], Beáta Scholtz [2] and Csongor Kiss [10]

1. Department of Operative Dentistry and Endodontics, Faculty of Dentistry, University of Debrecen, 4032 Debrecen, Hungary
2. Department of Biochemistry and Molecular Biology, Faculty of Medicine, University of Debrecen, 4032 Debrecen, Hungary; horvathjozsef21@gmail.com (J.H.); labiscsak.peter@med.unideb.hu (P.L.); jakob.bernadett@med.unideb.hu (B.M.); tozser@med.unideb.hu (J.T.); cseva@med.unideb.hu (É.C.); scholtz@med.unideb.hu (B.S.)
3. Department of Oral Pathology and Microbiology, Faculty of Dentistry and Institute of Pathology, University of Debrecen, 4032 Debrecen, Hungary; dezsob51@gmail.com
4. Department of Maxillofacial Surgery, University of Debrecen, 4032 Debrecen, Hungary; szabo.adrienn@dental.unideb.hu
5. Department of Oral Medicine, Faculty of Dentistry, University of Debrecen, 4032 Debrecen, Hungary; tar.ildiko@dental.unideb.hu
6. Department of Maxillofacial Surgery, University of Szeged, 6720 Szeged, Hungary; piffkojozsef@gmail.com (J.P.); jakus.petra.87@gmail.com (P.J.)
7. Department of Maxillofacial Surgery, Semmelweis University, 1085 Budapest, Hungary; barabas.jozsef@dent.semmelweis-univ.hu (J.B.); dr.barabas.peter@gmail.com (P.B.)
8. Department of Oral and Maxillofacial Surgery, University of Pécs, 7621 Pécs, Hungary; olasz.lajos@pte.hu (L.O.); kover.zsanett@pte.hu (Z.K.)
9. Department of Preventive Medicine, University of Debrecen, 4028 Debrecen, Hungary; sandor.janos@sph.unideb.hu
10. Department of Pediatric Hematology-Oncology, Faculty of Medicine, University of Debrecen, 4032 Debrecen, Hungary; kisscs@med.unideb.hu
* Correspondence: marton.ildiko@dental.unideb.hu; Tel.: +36-52-25-57-25

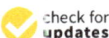

Received: 15 October 2019; Accepted: 9 November 2019; Published: 13 November 2019

Abstract: Salivary IL-6 mRNA was previously identified as a promising biomarker of oral squamous cell carcinoma (OSCC). We performed a multi-center investigation covering all geographic areas of Hungary. Saliva from 95 patients with OSCC and 80 controls, all Caucasian, were collected together with demographic and clinicopathological data. Salivary IL-6 mRNA was quantified by real-time quantitative PCR. Salivary IL-6 protein concentration was measured by enzyme-linked immune-sorbent assay. IL-6 protein expression in tumor samples was investigated by immunohistochemistry. Normalized salivary IL-6 mRNA expression values were significantly higher ($p < 0.001$) in patients with OSCC (mean ± SE: 3.301 ± 0.885) vs. controls (mean ± SE: 0.037 ± 0.012). Differences remained significant regardless of tumor stage and grade. AUC of the ROC curve was 0.9379 ($p < 0.001$; 95% confidence interval: 0.8973–0.9795; sensitivity: 0.945; specificity: 0.819). Salivary IL-6 protein levels were significantly higher ($p < 0.001$) in patients (mean ± SE: 70.98 ± 14.06 pg/mL), than in controls (mean ± SE: 12.45 ± 3.29). Specificity and sensitivity of IL-6 protein were less favorable than that of IL-6 mRNA. Salivary IL-6 mRNA expression was significantly associated with age and dental status. IL-6 manifestation was detected in tumor cells and tumor-infiltrating leukocytes, suggesting the presence of a paracrine loop of stimulation. Salivary IL-6 mRNA is one of the best performing and clinically relevant biomarkers of OSCC.

Keywords: salivary biomarkers; oral neoplasia; periodontal disease/periodontitis; smoking; ethanol consumption; real-time quantitative PCR; enzyme-linked immune-sorbent assay; immunohistochemistry

1. Introduction

Hungarian males and females exhibit the highest age-standardized rates both for the incidence and the mortality of oral cavity and pharyngeal cancers in Europe without substantial improvements in the last decades [1]. Frequently, oral squamous cell carcinoma (OSCC) is being diagnosed in advanced stages, i.e., stage III and IV, with long-term survival rates around 50% despite considerable progress in surgical methods, radio-, chemo-, and immunotherapy. In contrast, patients with early, i.e., stage I and II lesions, may experience recovery rates up to 80%. Unfortunately, with the exception of the gold standard procedure, tissue biopsy and histopathological analysis, there are no evidence-based, reliable, non-invasive methods for large-scale screening and early detection of OSCC [2,3].

The aim of the present investigation was to study the potential of salivary IL-6 mRNA and IL-6 protein as OSCC-related biomarkers. Saliva was chosen as a complex, informative body-fluid containing biomolecules that originate from multiple sources and may differentiate between healthy subjects and patients with OSCC. Application of advanced molecular methods resulted in the discovery of several candidate salivary proteins, metabolites, mRNAs, miRNAs, and circRNAs associated with OSCC. However, there has been a high degree of variation between results reported by different investigators with respect to the value of these biomolecules as biomarkers detected in patients of different geographic and ethnic backgrounds [4–10]. In addition, salivary levels of inflammatory cytokines, considered as one of the best performing molecular groups of OSCC biomarkers, may be confounded by the presence of oral inflammatory lesions [11–13].

Previously, we applied both targeted and high-throughput molecular methods to identify potentially useful mRNA and protein biomarkers in a small-scale single-institution pilot cohort of patients with OSCC and controls [12,13]. These pilot transcriptomic and proteomic investigations suggested that salivary IL-6 mRNA and protein may prove the best performing biomarkers of OSCC in the Hungarian population. Therefore, we investigated salivary IL-6 mRNA and IL-6 protein in a sample of patients with OSCC covering each geographic area of Hungary. To support the relevance of salivary IL-6 mRNA expression, we were looking for differences in salivary IL-6 protein concentrations of patients and controls and by detecting the expression of IL-6 protein in tumor cells and in tumor-infiltrating leukocytes (TIL). An additional objective was to analyze associations of salivary IL-6 mRNA and protein expression with age, sex, gingival inflammation status, smoking, and ethanol consumption habits in patients with OSCC.

2. Materials and Methods

2.1. Patients and Control Subjects

Between 2 May 2013 and 31 December 2015, 95 adult (>18 years) patients with OSCC, presenting a suitable saliva sample, were enrolled in a multi-centric investigation from four Hungarian sites: Faculty of Dentistry, University of Debrecen, Debrecen ("Debrecen Center"): 26 patients; Faculty of Dentistry, Scientific University of Szeged, Szeged ("Szeged Center"): 24 patients; Faculty of Dentistry, Scientific University of Pécs, Pécs ("Pécs Center"): 25 patients; and Faculty of Dentistry, Semmelweis University, Budapest ("Budapest Center"): 20 patients. Eighty age-matched adult controls, admitted for dental check-ups, were recruited from the same sites. Subjects with previous and present cancer, except for the present OSCC (patients), coexisting diabetes, autoimmune disorders, contagious diseases, and pregnancy were excluded.

The investigation was approved by the Institutional Review Board of the University of Debrecen (No. 3244–8/2011, No. 3722–2012) and by the Scientific and Research Ethics Committee, Medical Research Council, Hungary [(693/PI/12.) 45038-1/2012/EKU]. The Code of Ethics of the World Medical

Association and the ethical standards of the 2000 Revision of the Helsinki Declaration were respected. Signed informed consent was obtained from all participating subjects.

Examination of the oral cavity and the head and neck region was performed by a licensed dental and/or maxillofacial surgeon according to standard methods and criteria of the World Health Organization [14]. Tooth decay was characterized using the DMFT index by calculating the number of decayed (D), missing (M), and filled (F) teeth (T). Periodontal health was characterized by the gingival index (GI) [15]. Suspicious lesions were removed or biopsied, and OSCC was verified by histology investigating the hematoxylin- and eosin-stained slides. The histological differentiation grade of OSCC was defined according to the classification of the World Health Organization (WHO) [16]. The staging was performed according to the 8th edition of the TNM classification of the International Union Against Cancer [17]. Demographic and clinicopathological data, including age, sex, stage, and grade of OSCC, DMFT, and GI indices, were recorded. The stage and grade of OSCC lesions were not available from study subjects of the Pécs Center. Smoking and ethanol consumption habits were recorded from consenting subjects as precisely as possible. Based on the information obtained, we formed two groups in each category. Regarding smoking habits, we distinguished regular smokers and non-smokers/occasional smokers (<10 cigarettes/day). Regarding ethanol consumption habits, we formed two categories: people who consumed ethanol-containing beverages at least once a week vs. those who drank less than once a week.

2.2. Saliva Collection and Processing

Unstimulated saliva samples were collected between 9:00 and 11:00 a.m. Patients and controls refrained from eating, drinking, smoking, gum chewing, and performing oral hygiene measures for at least 60 min before sampling. A minimum of 5.0 mL saliva was collected from each participant. Samples were kept on ice throughout collection and processing. Samples were pushed five-times through a 19 g needle then filtered (Millex 25 mm Durapore PVDF 5 μm Sterile, Merck KGaA, Darmstadt, Germany). Three aliquots of 200 μL filtered saliva were mixed with 1 mL PAXgene® reagent in cryotubes, for immediate stabilization of salivary RNA (PAXgene® Blood RNA Tubes, BD Biosciences, Cat.No. 762165, BD Franklin Lakes, NJ, USA). Aliquots of 0.5 mL were pipetted from the remaining saliva filtrate into cryotubes, for ELISA (Cryopure tube, SARSTEDT, Cat.No. 72.380, Nümbrecht, Germany). The PAXgene®-stabilized and proteomic saliva samples were frozen within 60 min from collection and stored at −70 °C until processing.

2.3. Reverse Transcription and Real-Time Quantitative PCR (qPCR)

Salivary RNA was isolated with the Direct-zol™ RNA MiniPrep Plus Kit (Zymo research, Cat.No. R2072, Irvine, CA, USA) according to the manufacturer's instructions. RNA sample quality and concentration were characterized by Nanodrop spectrophotometry and by the Agilent 2100 Bioanalyzer system. Expression of IL-6 mRNA and two normalizing genes, GAPDH and ACTB, were quantified using qPCR with TaqMan® assays on a QuantStudio™ 12K Flex Real Time PCR System (Applied Biosystem®, Thermo Fisher Scientific, Waltham, MA, USA). Raw data analysis was performed using the ExpressionSuite Software v1.0.3 (Applied Biosystem®). Samples with a high standard deviation of replicates, or with only one replicate giving a signal in the qPCR assay were categorized as borderline, non-quantifiable-positive ones. Ct values of the latter samples were set uniformly to 39 for the calculations and statistical analysis.

For qPCR efficiency correction, raw Ct values of cDNA serial dilutions (from HeLa total RNA) were used to determine the slope of the assays, using the linear regression function of GraphPad Prism software (GraphPad Software, Inc., CA, USA). PCR efficiency values were calculated, Ct values were corrected, and data were normalized. qPCR efficiencies were as follows: IL-6 = 0.904, GAPDH = 0.814, ACTB = 1.03. Cutoff Ct values (limit of quantitation; LOQ) for each TaqMan® assay were also determined in these experiments. Detailed descriptions of RNA methods were provided as Supplementary data.

2.4. Enzyme-Linked Immune-Sorbent Assay (ELISA)

IL-6 protein concentration in saliva samples of patients and controls was determined in duplicates by the sandwich ELISA kit (Human ELISA Kit EK0410, Boster Biological Technology Co., Pleasanton, CA, USA) according to the manufacturer's instructions. Optical density was measured at 450 nm, and concentrations were calculated based on the recorded 7-point calibration curve. LOQ for IL-t6 protein concentration was 4.96 pg/mL.

2.5. Immunohistochemistry (IHC)

Sections obtained from 41 preexisting formalin-fixed and paraffin-embedded tissue blocks of patients with proven OSCC from the Debrecen Center were microscopically reviewed by an independent pathologist (BD). Since IHC labeling of preexisting tissue blocks did not interfere with salivary IL-6 mRNA and protein measurements, 15 samples from the previous pilot cohort were co-investigated with the 26 samples collected in the course of the present investigation to increase sample size [12,13]. Serial sections were used for the detection of IL-6 manifestation in tumor cells and TILs by IHC, as described in detail [18]. Briefly, mouse monoclonal antibodies (MoAb, clone 8H12; Invitrogen, Rockford, IL, USA) to IL-6 (8H12; Invitrogen; Thermo Fisher Scientific, Rockford, IL, USA), CD3, CD4, CD20, and CD163 (all from DAKO, Glostrup, Denmark) were used according to manufacturers' instructions. Peroxidase-conjugated anti-mouse secondary immunoglobulin was used with a peroxidase-based detection kit (DAKO, Glostrup, Denmark) and VIP or DAB chromogenic substrates (Vector Labs, Peterborough, UK) for visualization. Stained sections were digitalized using a Panoramic MIDI digital slide scanner (3D-Histech-Zeiss, Budapest, Hungary) equipped with a Hitachi (HV-F22CL) 3CCD camera. Image analysis was performed by the HistoQuant application of Panoramic viewer software 1.15.2 (3D-Histech, Budapest, Hungary) as described [19].

2.6. Statistical Analysis

Distribution of demographic characteristics and clinical parameters of patients and controls were described by mean values and standard deviations (SD) for continuous variables. One-way ANOVA for continuous and chi-square test for non-continuous variables were used to check for uneven distribution of patients' parameters between controls and cases. Statistical computation was carried out by IBM SPSS Statistics version 20 (IBM SPSS Statistics for Windows, Version 20.0, Armonk, NY, USA).

In describing the expression of IL-6 mRNA and IL-6 protein, mean values and standard errors (SE) were computed. Differences between patients and controls were assessed with GraphPad Prism, using the Mann-Whitney U-test on the efficiency-corrected, normalized IL-6 mRNA expression values, and IL-6 protein concentration values.

Receiver Operating Characteristic (ROC) curve analysis was carried out on the same data with GraphPad Prism to evaluate the discrimination properties of IL-6 mRNA and IL-6 protein, and the area under the curve (AUC) was determined.

Multivariate linear regression models were applied to investigate the influence of patients' age, sex, DMFT score, GI score, smoking, and ethanol consumption on IL-6 mRNA and IL-6 protein concentrations. Before modeling, IL-6 mRNA and IL-6 protein concentrations were ln-transformed because of these parameters showed right-tailed distribution. The normal distribution of ln transformed values was checked by the Kolmogorov-Smirnov test. Results were described by linear regression coefficients with the corresponding p-values. Statistical computation was carried out by IBM SPSS Statistics version 20.

3. Results

3.1. Characteristics of Study Participants

Demographic and clinicopathological characterization of 95 patients with newly diagnosed and histologically-verified OSCC and 80 age-matched controls were summarized in Table 1. There were more males ($N = 60$) than females ($N = 35$) among patients with OSCC, resulting in a significant difference in sex distribution between the patient and control groups. The patient group was characterized by significantly higher DMFT scores than the group of controls. Smoking and ethanol consumption were significantly more frequent among patients than controls. Both IL-6 mRNA and IL-6 protein determination were successfully performed in 53 patient samples. Twenty-one and 21 samples, each, from different patients were suitable for either IL-6 mRNA or IL-6 protein measurements. In the case of the 80 controls, the number of successful salivary analyses were as follows, IL-6 mRNA and IL-6 protein: 55, IL-6 mRNA only: 9, and IL-6 protein: only 16 (Table S1: Demographic, cliniccpathological characterization, and IL-6 mRNA and IL-6 protein levels of individual patients with OSCC and controls).

Table 1. Demographic and clinicopathological characterization of patients with oral squamous cell carcinoma (OSCC) and control subjects.

	-	Patients (N = 95)	Controls (N = 80)	P
Sex	Male	60 (63%)	30 (37%)	0.004 *
	Female	35 (37%)	50 (63%)	
Age	(years; mean ± SD)	61.7 ± 9.8	61.7 ± 9.2	0.982 **
OSCC stage				
	St I	14 (20%)	–	na ***
N = 70	St II	22 (31%)	–	na ***
	St III	13 (19%)	–	na***
	St IV	21 (30%)	–	na ***
Histological grade				
	G1	17 (24%)	–	na ***
N = 70	G2	42 (60%)	–	na ***
	G3	11 (16%)	–	na ***
DMFT	(N; mean ± SD)	64; 27.6 ± 6.4	47; 24.8 ± 6.9	0.011 **
GI	(N; mean ± SD)	36; 0.53 ± 0.49	41; 0.42 ± 0.34	0.79 **
Ethanol consumption	at least once a week	46 (48%)	14 (30%)	0.035 *
	less than once a week	49 (52%)	33 (70%)	
Smoking	regular smoking	62 (65%)	8 (17%)	<0.001 *
	non-smoker or occasional smoker	33 (35%)	40 (83%)	

N = number of patients * chi-square test; ** t-test; *** not applicable.

3.2. Salivary IL-6 mRNA and IL-6 Protein Expression

Saliva samples of 74/95 patients and 64/80 controls were suitable for qPCR. The majority of saliva samples from patients were positive for IL-6 mRNA. Initially, there were 18 samples with no quantifiable results. Reverse transcription and qPCR of these cases were repeated, resulting in 71 quantifiable results of 74 IL-6 mRNA samples from patients with OSCC. In contrast, 46 of 64 control samples were non-quantifiable (36 negative, and 10 borderline positive samples) for IL-6 mRNA expression, even in the repeated measurements. Normalized salivary IL-6 mRNA expression values were significantly higher in the group of patients with OSCC than in controls. The difference remained significant when subgroups of patients with different stages and grades were compared with controls (Table 2, Figure 1A). There were no significant differences in IL-6 mRNA expression between subgroups of patients with different stages and grades (data not shown). To test the sensitivity and specificity of salivary IL-6 mRNA as a diagnostic biomarker for OSCC, an ROC curve analysis was performed, and the AUC was calculated. The AUC for IL-6 mRNA was 0.9379 ($p < 0.001$; 95% confidence interval: 0.8973–0.9795; sensitivity: 0.945; specificity: 0.819) (Figure 1C).

Table 2. Differential expression of IL6 mRNA and IL6 protein in the saliva of patients with OSCC and controls.

	IL-6 mRNA Normalized Values				IL-6 Protein [pg/mL]			
Sample	N	mean	SE	p *	N	mean	SE	p *
OSCC								
St I-II	31	1.634	0.400	<0.001	30	59.72	18.09	<0.001
St III-IV	23	23.694	19.850	<0.001	28	102.44	28.22	<0.001
G1	9	1.440	0.501	<0.001	16	39.08	10.92	0.005
G2	34	16.327	13.550	<0.001	35	102.56	26.24	<0.001
G3	11	2.505	1.540	<0.001	7	63.58	22.45	0.010
Total	74	3.301	0.885	<0.001	74	70.98	14.06	<0.001
Control	64	0.037	0.012		71	12.45	3.29	

* Statistical comparison (Mann-Whitney U-test) of indicated groups of patient and control samples. There were no significant differences either in IL6 mRNA or IL6 protein expression between different subgroups of patients according to tumor stages and grades.

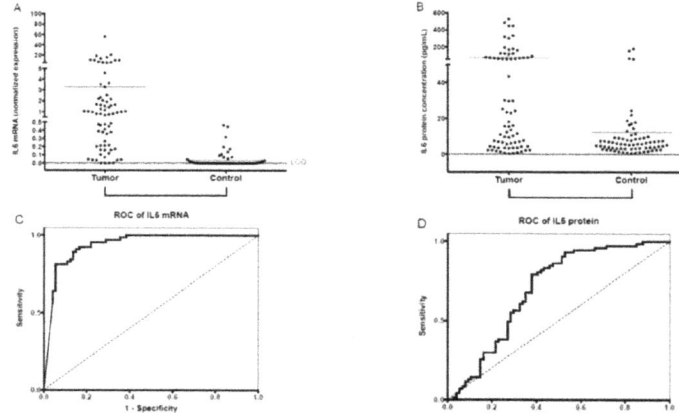

Figure 1. Salivary IL-6 mRNA and IL-6 protein expression. Expression of normalized salivary IL-6 mRNA (**A**) and salivary IL-6 protein (**B**) in patients with OSCC and controls. The horizontal lines indicate the mean. The p values are derived from the Mann-Whitney U test. Differences between Tumor and Control groups proved significant at $p < 0.001$ for both salivary IL-6 mRNA normalized values and for salivary IL-6 protein concentrations ($p < 0.05$ was considered significant). Dotted lines indicate the limit of quantification (LOQ). Receiver operating characteristic (ROC) curves for diagnostic ability of IL-6 mRNA (**C**) and protein (**D**) levels in saliva for OSCC. AUC for IL-6 mRNA = 0.9379 ($p < 0.001$; 95% confidence interval: 0.8973–0.9795; sensitivity: 0.945; specificity: 0.819); AUC for IL-6 protein = 0.6981 ($p < 0.0001$; 95% confidence interval: 0.6105–0.7858; sensitivity: 0.622; specificity: 0.789).

IL-6 protein concentration was measured in 74 suitable salivary samples of 95 patients and in 71/80 controls. Patients with OSCC, both the total patient group and subgroups of patients according to stages and grades, had statistically significantly higher IL-6 concentrations than controls (Table 2, Figure 1B). There were no significant differences in IL-6 protein concentrations of subgroups of patients with different stages and grades. There was a partial overlap between the distribution of the salivary IL-6 protein concentration of the patient and the control groups (Figure 1B). Using ROC analysis, salivary IL-6 protein concentration successfully identified patients with OSCC. The AUC for IL-6 protein was 0.6981 ($p < 0.0001$; 95% confidence interval: 0.6105–0.7858; sensitivity: 0.622; specificity: 0.789) (Figure 1D).

According to the multivariate linear regression analysis, the age and DMFT score had significant associations with ln transformed IL-6 mRNA expression levels. Sex, GI scores, alcohol consumption, and smoking exhibited no statistically significant association either with salivary IL-6 RNA or IL-6 protein expression (Table 3).

Table 3. Associations between demographic variables, gingival inflammation status, ethanol consumption, and smoking habits and ln-transformed salivary levels of IL-6 mRNA and IL-6 protein according to multivariate linear regression analysis.

		In Transformed IL-6 mRNA		In Transformed IL-6 Protein	
		Adjusted linear regression coefficient	p-value	Adjusted linear regression coefficient	p-value
Sex	female/male	−0.181	0.1	−0.159	0.11
Age	**Year**	**0.234**	**0.037**	0.174	0.094
DMFT		**0.234**	**0.037**	0.174	0.094
Gingival index		0.094	0.488	0.201	0.1
Alcohol consumption at least once a week/less than once a week		0.561	0.07	−0.1	0.375
Smoking regular smoking non-smoker or Occasional smoker		−0.134	0.232	0.005	0.959

Significant associations are indicated in bold characters.

3.3. IL-6 Protein Expression in OSCC Tumor Tissue

We performed an IHC investigation of the neoplastic lesions so as to see if the IL-6 mRNA and protein detected in the saliva of patients with OSCC might be produced by cells in the tumor tissue. We detected a positive IL-6 reaction in 28/41 (68%) samples. In 16/41 samples, neoplastic cells were stained positively, and in 26/41 samples, there were detectable IL-6 protein expression in TILs (Figure 2). TILs consisted mostly of neutrophil granulocytes, CD163-positive macrophages, and CD3-positive T-lymphocytes. Occasionally, CD20-positive B-lymphocytes, plasma cells, and eosinophil granulocytes were found. CD4-positive T-cells predominated over CD8-positive T-cells. The CD4:CD8 ratio was 2:1 in 30/41 (73%) of cases. We noted a CD4:CD8 inversion (CD4:CD8 < 1:2) in 5/41 (12%) cases without signs of tumor cell destruction.

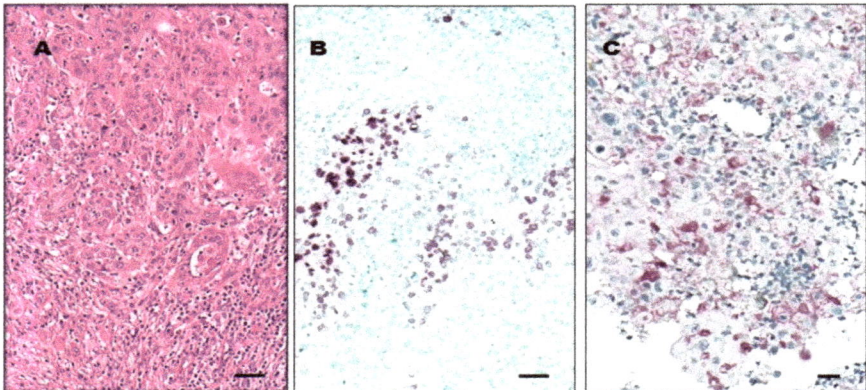

Figure 2. IL-6 protein expression in OSCC tumor tissue. Images from a representative tissue sample exhibiting OSCC with moderate differentiation grade (G2). (**A**) Abundant peri- and intratumoral tumor-infiltrating leukocytes (TILs) surrounding and intermixed with tumor cells (hematoxylin-eosin staining). (**B**) A region of a representative tumor sample showing many IL-6-positive TILs, whereas cancer cells are negative for IL-6 staining. (**C**) Another region of the same representative tumor sample with large squamous carcinoma cells exhibiting IL-6 positivity. Original magnification for all three images is 20×. Horizontal bars indicate 20 µm. Images (B) and (C) represent the immunohistochemistry (IHC) reaction using the peroxidase-based technique with VIP chromogen, as described in Materials and Methods.

4. Discussion

The aim of the present investigation was to validate salivary IL-6 mRNA and protein as a diagnostic biomarker of OSCC. Saliva samples from patients with histologically proven, newly diagnosed OSCC were collected from tertiary treatment centers representing each geographic region of Hungary. The age distribution of patients was similar to previously reported Hungarian regional and nation-wide epidemiologic data. The predominance of female patients with 37% and the prevalence of advanced patients (stage 3 and 4: 62%) in the present investigation was more expressed than observed previously [1,12,20,21]. Although the distribution pattern of histological differentiation grades (G2 > G1 > G3) was similar as that reported in a previous North-Eastern Hungarian cohort, the ratio of less differentiated grades (G2 and G3) was slightly higher but the same as in the preliminary institutional pilot investigation [12,20].

Salivary IL-6 was chosen as the potentially best-performing biomarker from 9 mRNA and 14 protein molecules tested in a small-scale pilot cohort of patients from one of the participating centers (Debrecen) [12,13]. Results on quantitatively determined salivary IL-6 mRNA transcripts have not yet been published prior to our previous pilot cohort and the present multi-center study investigating the largest number of patients with OSCC. Earlier only one study reported on the expression of salivary IL-6 mRNA in patients with OSCC; however, the level of expression was not quantified [22]. We found IL-6 mRNA transcripts by qPCR in 71 of 74 saliva samples of patients with OSCC. In contrast, only 18 of 64 control saliva samples contained quantifiable levels of IL-6 mRNA transcripts, and there was a statistically significant difference in the expression levels of normalized IL-6 mRNA transcripts between patients and controls. With an AUC value of 0.9379 of the ROC curve, IL-6 mRNA is one of the best-performing salivary OSCC biomarkers reported so far [10,23–25].

At the protein level, salivary IL-6 was reported most consistently to distinguish between patients with OSCC and controls with different geographic and ethnic backgrounds. Results with other salivary protein biomarkers were found less coherent [11]. We observed significantly higher IL-6 protein concentrations in the saliva of patients with OSCC vs. controls; however, there was a partial overlap between the distribution of salivary IL-6 concentrations of patients and controls, resulting in a less favorable AUC value of the ROC curve than with salivary IL-6 mRNA. Similar salivary IL-6 concentrations to our results were observed in patients with OSCC by other investigators [4,26–35]. The attempt at normalizing salivary IL-6 protein concentration for salivary total protein concentration abolished the significant difference of salivary IL-6 manifestation observed between patients and controls (data not shown). IL-6 is a low-abundance salivary protein with a concentration in the pg/mL range, whereas salivary total protein concentration is in the mg/mL range and the low signal-to-noise ratio might obscure differences [32]. Moreover, salivary albumin, a high-abundance salivary protein, was reported to correlate with OSCC, similar to IL-6, which may further compromise normalized results [35]. In addition to OSCC, salivary IL-6 protein concentration was investigated in oral premalignant lesions (OPML). The majority of investigators found significantly increased salivary IL-6 protein concentrations in patients with OPML when compared to controls, although the concentration was less excessively elevated in OPML than in OSCC samples [26,34,36,37]. In contrast, Brailo et al. found significantly elevated IL-6 protein concentrations in salivary samples from patients with OSCC but not with OPML [31], suggesting that further studies are requested before establishing a discriminatory role of salivary IL-6 protein between OSCC and OPML. Since data on salivary IL-6 mRNA in patients with OPML are lacking, we can either confirm or refute if salivary IL-6 mRNA, although remarkably sensitive for OSCC, would be proven specific for OSCC as compared to OPML.

Few groups investigated salivary IL-6 expression in association with various tumor stages and differentiation grades. In our study, differences both in salivary IL-6 mRNA and protein expression levels remained significant when comparing subgroups of patients with OSCC according to the stage and grade of their disease with controls, and there were no differences between distinct subgroups of patients. Similar results were reported by Sato et al. and Lisa Cheng et al. [29,32]. Three other groups observed higher salivary IL-6 concentration in patients with advanced lesions [27,32,33].

Conflicting results were reported on the potential influence of age, sex, smoking, and ethanol consumption habits on salivary IL-6 protein concentration in patients with OSCC [27,29,31,33,36]. Using linear regression analysis, we found significant associations between age and DMFT scores and salivary IL-6 mRNA expression confirming the results of our previous pilot studies, suggesting the influence of oral health on salivary OSCC biomarkers [12,13]. Yet, the separation between salivary mRNA levels of patients with and without OSCC is robust enough to maintain its value as an OSCC biomarker. Sex, smoking, and ethanol consumption did not bias the expression of either salivary IL-6 mRNA or IL-6 protein.

In a search for the source of elevated salivary IL-6 levels in patients with OSCC, we investigated the expression of IL-6 protein in the tumor tissue. In the majority of cases, tumor cells, and TILs were positive for IL-6 staining. Similar observations were reported in one publication [38]. These results, together with experimental evidence, suggest that a paracrine loop of stimulation may exist between neoplastic and nonmalignant cells of the tumor microenvironment [39,40]. The positive feedback loop of stimulation may explain the significant upregulation of salivary IL6 expression in patients with OSCC both at the mRNA and protein level when compared to controls. Thus, the IL-6-IL-6 receptor interaction may offer therapeutic targets in OSCC [41].

In conclusion, salivary IL-6 mRNA is a robust biomarker for OSCC in the Hungarian population in comparison with tumor-free control persons. However, caution is warranted before claiming the specificity of this biomarker without investigating salivary IL-6 mRNA in patients with OPML. Further investigations, involving patients from different ethnic groups and geographic regions may prove the value of quantitative salivary IL-6 mRNA expression as a general OSCC biomarker. The relevance of salivary IL-6 mRNA in OSCC was supported by the significantly elevated salivary IL-6 protein concentration in patients with OSCC vs. controls. Moreover, intratumor IL-6 production both by tumor cells and TILs, detected by IHC, may serve as a likely source of salivary IL-6 mRNA and protein in patients with OSCC.

Supplementary Materials: The following are available online at http://www.mdpi.com/2077-0383/8/11/1958/s1, Table S1: Demographic, clinicopathological characterization and IL-6 mRNA and IL-6 protein levels of individual patients with OSCC and controls.

Author Contributions: Conceptualization, I.J.M., J.T., J.S., B.S. and C.K.; data curation, J.S., B.S. and C.K.; formal analysis, P.L., B.M., J.S. and C.K.; funding acquisition, I.J.M.; investigation, I.J.M., J.H., P.L., B.M., B.D., A.S., I.T., J.P., P.J., J.B., P.B., L.O., Z.K., É.C. and C.K.; methodology, I.J.M., J.H., P.L., B.M., B.D., É.C. and B.S.; project administration, I.J.M., É.C., B.S. and C.K.; resources, I.J.M., I.T., J.P., J.B., L.O., J.T., É.C., B.S. and C.K.; software, J.S.; supervision, I.J.M., J.P., J.B. and L.O.; validation, I.J.M. and B.S.; visualization, B.D., É.C. and B.S.; writing—original draft, I.J.M., B.D., J.T., É.C., B.S. and C.K.; writing—review and editing, B.D., É.C., B.S. and C.K.

Funding: This work was supported by the Hungarian Scientific Research Fund (OTKA) 105034, by the János Bolyai Scholarship of the Hungarian Academy of Sciences, and by ÚNKP-18-4-DE-436.

Acknowledgments: The technical assistance of Hajnalka J. Tóth is acknowledged.

Conflicts of Interest: The authors declare no conflict of interest.

References

1. Diz, P.; Meleti, M.; Diniz-Freitas, M.; Vescovi, P.; Warnakulasuriya, S.; Johnson, N.W.; Kerr, A.R. Oral and pharyngeal cancer in Europe: Incidence, mortality and trends as presented to the Global Oral Cancer Forum. *Trans. Res. Oral Oncol.* **2017**, *2*, 1–13. [CrossRef]
2. Zhang, H.; Dziegielewski, P.T.; Biron, V.L.; Szudek, J.; Al-Qahatani, K.H.; O'Connell, D.A. Survival outcomes of patients with advanced oral cavity squamous cell carcinoma treated with multimodal therapy: A multi-institutional analysis. *J. Otolaryngol. Head Neck Surg.* **2013**, *42*, 30. [CrossRef] [PubMed]
3. Carreras-Torras, C.; Gay-Escoda, C. Techniques for early diagnosis of oral squamous cell carcinoma: Systematic review. *Med. Oral Patol. Oral Cir. Bucal.* **2015**, *20*, e305–e315. [CrossRef] [PubMed]
4. SahebJamee, M.; Eslami, M.; AtarbashiMoghadam, F.; Sarafnejad, A. Salivary concentration of TNFalpha, IL1 alpha, IL6, and IL8 in oral squamous cell carcinoma. *Med. Oral Patol. Oral Cir. Bucal.* **2008**, *13*, E292–E295. [PubMed]
5. Wu, J.Y.; Yi, C.; Chung, H.R.; Wang, D.J.; Chang, W.C.; Lee, S.Y.; Lin, C.T.; Yang, Y.C.; Yang, W.C. Potential biomarkers in saliva for oral squamous cell carcinoma. *Oral Oncol.* **2010**, *46*, 226–231. [CrossRef]
6. Panta, P.; Venna, V.R. Salivary RNA signatures in oral cancer detection. *Anal. Cell. Pathol.* **2014**, *2014*, 450629. [CrossRef]
7. Khan, R.S.; Khurshid, Z.; Akhbar, S.; Faraz Moin, S. Advances of Salivary Proteomics in Oral Squamous Cell Carcinoma (OSCC) Detection: An Update. *Proteomes* **2016**, *4*, 41. [CrossRef]
8. Radhika, T.; Jeddy, N.; Nithya, S.; Muthumeenakshi, R.M. Salivary biomarkers in oral squamous cell carcinoma—An insight. *J. Oral Biol. Craniofac. Res.* **2016**, *6*, S51–S54. [CrossRef]
9. Lohavanichbutr, P.; Zhang, Y.; Wang, P.; Gu, H.; Nagana Gowda, G.A.; Djukovic, D.; Buas, M.F.; Raftery, D.; Chen, C. Salivary metabolite profiling distinguishes patients with oral cavity squamous cell carcinoma from normal controls. *PLoS ONE* **2018**, *13*, e0204249. [CrossRef]
10. Zhao, S.Y.; Wang, J.; Ouyang, S.B.; Huang, Z.K.; Liao, L. Salivary Circular RNAs Hsa_Circ_0001874 and Hsa_Circ_0001971 as Novel Biomarkers for the Diagnosis of Oral Squamous Cell Carcinoma. *Cell. Physiol. Biochem.* **2018**, *47*, 2511–2521. [CrossRef]
11. Sahibzada, H.A.; Khurshid, Z.; Khan, R.S.; Naseem, M.; Siddique, K.M.; Mali, M.; Zafar, M.S. Salivary IL-8, IL-6 and TNF-α as potential diagnostic biomarkers for oral cancer. *Diagnostics* **2017**, *7*, 21. [CrossRef] [PubMed]
12. Horváth, J.; Szabó, A.; Tar, I.; Dezső, B.; Kiss, C.; Márton, I.; Scholtz, B. Oral health may affect the performance of mRNA-based saliva biomarkers for oral squamous cell cancer. *Pathol. Oncol. Res.* **2018**, *24*, 833–842. [CrossRef] [PubMed]
13. Csősz, É.; Lábiscsák, P.; Kalló, G.; Márkus, B.; Emri, M.; Szabó, A.; Tar, I.; Tőzsér, J.; Kiss, C.; Márton, I. Proteomics investigation of OSCC-specific salivary biomarkers in a Hungarian population highlights the importance of identification of population-tailored biomarkers. *PLoS ONE* **2017**, *12*, e0177282. [CrossRef] [PubMed]
14. World Health Organization. *Oral Health Surveys: Basic Methods*, 4th ed.; World Health Organization: Geneva, Switzerland, 1997.
15. Lang, N.P.; Corbet, E.F. Periodontal diagnosis in daily practice. *Int. Dent. J.* **1995**, *45*, 3–15. [PubMed]
16. Pindborg, J.J.; Reichart, P.A.; Smith, C.J.; Van der Waal, I. *Histological Typing of Cancer and Precancer of the Oral Mucosa. WHO International Histological Classification of Tumours*, 2nd ed.; Springer: Berlin, Germany, 1997.

17. Sobin, L.H.; Gospodarowitz, M.K.; Wittekind, C. Head and Neck Tumours: Lip and oral cavity. In *TNM Classification of Malignant Tumours*, 7th ed.; Wiley-Blackwell: Chichester, UK, 2010; pp. 25–29.
18. Tsakiris, I.; Torocsik, D.; Gyongyosi, A.; Dozsa, A.; Szatmari, I.; Szanto, A.; Soos, G.; Nemes, Z.; Igali, L.; Marton, I.; et al. Carboxypeptidase-M is regulated by lipids and CSFs in macrophages and dendritic cells and expressed selectively in tissue granulomas and foam cells. *Lab. Investig.* **2012**, *92*, 345–361. [CrossRef] [PubMed]
19. Szabó, K.; Papp, G.; Dezso, B.; Zeher, M. The histopathology of labial salivary glands in primary Sjögren' syndrome: Focusing on follicular helper T cells in the inflammatory infiltrates. *Mediators Inflamm.* **2014**, *2014*, 631787. [CrossRef]
20. Nemes, J.A.; Redl, P.; Boda, R.; Kiss, C.; Márton, I.J. Oral cancer report from Northeastern Hungary. *Pathol. Oncol. Res.* **2008**, *14*, 85–92. [CrossRef]
21. Németh, Z.; Turi, K.; Léhner, G.; Veres, D.S.; Csurgay, K. The prognostic role of age in oral cancer. A clinical study. *Magy. Onkol.* **2013**, *57*, 166–172. (In Hungarian)
22. St John, M.A.; Li, Y.; Zhou, X.; Denny, P.; Ho, C.M.; Montemagno, C.; Shi, W.; Qi, F.; Wu, B.; Sinha, U.; et al. Interleukin 6 and interleukin 8 as potential biomarkers for oral cavity and oropharyngeal squamous cell carcinoma. *Arch. Otolaryngol. Head Neck Surg.* **2004**, *130*, 929–935. [CrossRef]
23. Brinkmann, O.; Kastratovic, D.A.; Dimitrijevic, M.V.; Konstantinovic, V.S.; Jelovac, D.B.; Antic, J.; Nesic, V.S.; Markovic, S.Z.; Martinovic, Z.R.; Akin, D.; et al. Oral squamous cell carcinoma detection by salivary biomarkers in Serbian population. *Oral Oncol.* **2011**, *47*, 51–55. [CrossRef]
24. Gai, C.; Camussi, F.; Broccoletti, R.; Gambino, A.; Cabras, M.; Molinaro, L.; Carossa, S.; Camussi, G.; Arduino, P.G. Salivary extracellular vesicle-associated miRNAs as potential biomarkers in oral squamous cell carcinoma. *BMC Cancer* **2018**, *18*, 439. [CrossRef] [PubMed]
25. Feng, Y.; Li, Q.; Chen, J.; Yi, P.; Xu, X.; Fan, Y.; Cui, B.; Yu, Y.; Li, X.; Du, Y.; et al. Salivary protease spectrum biomarkers of oral cancer. *Int. J. Oral Sci.* **2019**, *11*, 7. [CrossRef] [PubMed]
26. Rhodus, N.L.; Ho, V.; Miller, C.S.; Myers, S.; Ondrey, F. NF-kappaB dependent cytokine levels in saliva of patients with oral paraneoplastic lesions and oral squamous cell carcinoma. *Cancer Detect. Prev.* **2005**, *29*, 42–45. [CrossRef] [PubMed]
27. Duffy, S.A.; Taylor, J.M.; Terrell, J.E.; Islam, M.; Li, Y.; Wolf, G.T.; Teknos, T.N. Interleukin-6 predicts recurrence and survival among head and neck cancer patients. *Cancer* **2008**, *113*, 750–757. [CrossRef] [PubMed]
28. Katakura, A.; Kamiyama, I.; Takano, N.; Shibahara, T.; Muramatsu, T.; Ishihara, K.; Takagi, R.; Shouno, T. Comparison of salivary cytokine levels in oral cancer patients and healthy subjects. *Bull. Tokyo Dent. Coll.* **2007**, *48*, 199–203. [CrossRef] [PubMed]
29. Sato, J.; Goto, J.; Murata, T.; Kitamori, S.; Yamazaki, Y.; Satoh, A.; Kitagawa, Y. Changes in saliva interleukin-6 levels in patients with oral squamous cell carcinoma. *Oral Surg. Oral Med. Oral Pathol. Oral Radiol. Endod.* **2010**, *110*, 330–336. [CrossRef] [PubMed]
30. Korostoff, A.; Reder, L.; Masood, R.; Sinha, U.K. The role of salivary cytokine biomarkers in tongue cancer invasion and mortality. *Oral Oncol.* **2011**, *47*, 282–287. [CrossRef]
31. Brailo, V.; Vucicevic-Boras, V.; Lukac, J.; Biocina-Lukenda, D.; Zilic-Alajbeg, I.; Milenovic, A.; Balija, M. Salivary and serum interleukin 1 beta, interleukin 6 and tumor necrosis factor alpha in patients with leukoplakia and oral cancer. *Med. Oral Patol. Oral Cir. Bucal* **2012**, *17*, e10–e15. [CrossRef]
32. Lisa Cheng, Y.S.; Jordan, L.; Gorugantula, L.M.; Schneiderman, E.; Chen, H.S.; Rees, T. Salivary interleukin-6 and -8 in patients with oral cancer and patients with chronic oral inflammatory diseases. *J. Periodontol.* **2014**, *85*, 956–965. [CrossRef]
33. Arduino, P.G.; Menegatti, E.; Cappello, N.; Martina, E.; Gardino, N.; Tanteri, C.; Cavallo, F.; Scully, C.; Broccoletti, R. Possible role for interleukins as biomarkers for mortality and recurrence in oral cancer. *Int. J. Biol. Markers* **2015**, *30*, e262–e266. [CrossRef]
34. Panneer Selvam, N.; Sadaksharam, J. Salivary interleukin-6 in the detection of oral cancer and precancer. *Asia. Pac. J. Clin. Oncol.* **2015**, *11*, 236–241. [CrossRef]
35. Rao, M.; Ramesh, A.; Adapa, S.; Thomas, B.; Shetty, J. Correlation of salivary levels of interleukin-6 and albumin with oral squamous cell carcinoma. *J. Health Res. Rev.* **2016**, *3*, 11–14. [CrossRef]
36. Juretic, M.; Cerovic, R.; Belusic-Gobic, M.; Brekalo Prso, I.; Kqiku, L.; Spalj, S.; Pezelj-Ribaric, S. Salivary levels of TNF-α and IL-6 in patients with oral premalignant and malignant lesions. *Folia Biol.* **2013**, *59*, 99–102.
37. Dikova, V.R.; Principe, S.; Bagan, J.V. Salivary inflammatory proteins in patients with oral potentially malignant disorders. *J. Clin. Exp. Dent.* **2019**, *11*, e659–e664. [CrossRef] [PubMed]

38. Jinno, T.; Kawano, S.; Maruse, Y.; Matsubara, R.; Goto, Y.; Sakamoto, T.; Hashiguchi, Y.; Kaneko, N.; Tanaka, H.; Kitamura, R. Increased expression of interleukin-6 predicts poor response to chemoradiotherapy and unfavorable prognosis in oral squamous cell carcinoma. *Oncol. Rep.* **2015**, *33*, 2161–2168. [CrossRef] [PubMed]
39. Yamamoto, T.; Kimura, T.; Ueta, E.; Tatemoto, Y.; Osaki, T. Characteristic cytokine generation patterns in cancer cells and infiltrating lymphocytes in oral squamous cell carcinomas and the influence of chemoradiation combined with immunotherapy on these patterns. *Oncology* **2003**, *64*, 407–415. [CrossRef]
40. Petruzzi, M.N.; Cherubini, K.; Salum, F.G.; de Figueiredo, M.A. Role of tumour-associated macrophages in oral squamous cells carcinoma progression: An update on current knowledge. *Diagn. Pathol.* **2017**, *12*, 32. [CrossRef]
41. Rossi, J.F.; Lu, Z.Y.; Jourdan, M.; Klein, B. Interleukin-6 as a therapeutic target. *Clin. Cancer Res.* **2015**, *21*, 1248–1257. [CrossRef]

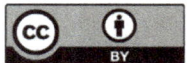

© 2019 by the authors. Licensee MDPI, Basel, Switzerland. This article is an open access article distributed under the terms and conditions of the Creative Commons Attribution (CC BY) license (http://creativecommons.org/licenses/by/4.0/).

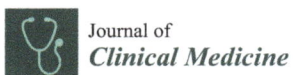

Review

Association of Salivary Human Papillomavirus Infection and Oral and Oropharyngeal Cancer: A Meta-Analysis

Óscar Rapado-González [1,2,3], Cristina Martínez-Reglero [4], Ángel Salgado-Barreira [4], Almudena Rodríguez-Fernández [5], Santiago Aguín-Losada [6], Luis León-Mateos [6], Laura Muinelo-Romay [2,3], Rafael López-López [3,6,*] and María Mercedes Suarez-Cunqueiro [1,3,7,*]

1. Department of Surgery and Medical-Surgical Specialties, Medicine and Dentistry School, Universidade de Santiago de Compostela (USC), 15782 Santiago de Compostela, Spain; oscar.rapado@rai.usc.es
2. Liquid Biopsy Analysis Unit, Translational Medical Oncology (Oncomet), Health Research Institute of Santiago (IDIS), 15706 Santiago de Compostela, Spain; lmuirom@gmail.com
3. Centro de Investigación Biomédica en Red en Cáncer (CIBERONC), Instituto de Salud Carlos III, 28029 Madrid, Spain
4. Methodology and Statistics Unit, Galicia Sur Health Research Institute (IISGS), 36312 Vigo, Spain; cristina.martinez@iisgaliciasur.es (C.M.-R.); angel.salgado.barreira@sergas.es (Á.S.-B.)
5. Department of Preventive and Public Health, Universidade de Santiago de Compostela (USC), 15782 Santiago de Compostela, Spain; almudena.rodríguez@usc.es
6. Translational Medical Oncology (Oncomet), Health Research Institute of Santiago (IDIS), Complexo Hospitalario Universitario de Santiago de Compostela (SERGAS), 15706 Santiago de Compostela, Spain; lanfear22@hotmail.com (S.A.-L.); Luis.Angel.Leon.Mateos@sergas.es (L.L.-M.)
7. Translational Medical Oncology (Oncomet), Health Research Institute of Santiago (IDIS), 15706 Santiago de Compostela, Spain
* Correspondence: rafa.lopez.lopez@gmail.com (R.L.-L.); mariamercedes.suarez@usc.es (M.M.S.-C.); Tel.: +34-981-95-14-70 (R.L-L.); +34-881-812-437 (M.M.S.-C.)

Received: 31 March 2020; Accepted: 26 April 2020; Published: 29 April 2020

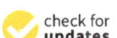

Abstract: Background. Human papillomavirus (HPV) infection has been recognized as an important risk factor in cancer. The purpose of this systematic review and meta-analysis was to determine the prevalence and effect size of association between salivary HPV DNA and the risk of developing oral and oropharyngeal cancer. Methods. A systematic literature search of PubMed, EMBASE, Web of Science, LILACS, Scopus and the Cochrane Library was performed, without language restrictions or specified start date. Pooled data were analyzed by calculating odds ratios (ORs) and 95% confidence intervals (CIs). Quality assessment was performed using the Newcastle–Ottawa Scale (NOS). Results. A total of 1672 studies were screened and 14 met inclusion criteria for the meta-analysis. The overall prevalence of salivary HPV DNA for oral and oropharyngeal carcinoma was 43.2%, and the prevalence of salivary HPV16 genotype was 27.5%. Pooled results showed a significant association between salivary HPV and oral and oropharyngeal cancer (OR = 4.94; 2.82–8.67), oral cancer (OR = 2.58; 1.67–3.99) and oropharyngeal cancer (OR = 17.71; 6.42–48.84). Significant associations were also found between salivary HPV16 and oral and oropharyngeal cancer (OR = 10.07; 3.65–27.82), oral cancer (OR = 2.95; 1.23–7.08) and oropharyngeal cancer (OR = 38.50; 22.43–66.07). Conclusions. Our meta-analysis demonstrated the association between salivary HPV infection and the incidence of oral and oropharyngeal cancer indicating its value as a predictive indicator.

Keywords: human papillomavirus; oral cancer; oropharyngeal cancer; saliva; meta-analysis

1. Introduction

Human papillomavirus (HPV) infection has been recognized as an important risk factor in a subset of head and neck squamous cell carcinomas, independently of traditional risk factors such as tobacco or alcohol use [1,2]. Globally, around 38,000 cases of head and neck cancer are attributed to the HPV infection. Of these, around 76% are cases of oropharynx cancer, 12% of oral cavity cancer and 10% of larynx cancer [3]. Currently, it is well known that HPV-status determines the molecular landscape of these tumors and their clinical evolution, with a better prognosis and response to therapy being found in HPV-positive patients [4,5].

HPVs are small, non-enveloped, close-circular, double-stranded DNA viruses of approximately 8000 base-pairs which present a specific tissue tropism infecting epithelial cells of the skin and mucosae of the anogenital and upper aero-digestive tract [6]. More than 200 different HPV types have been identified and classified into low-risk and high-risk according to their oncogenic potential. In this sense, high-risk HPV (HR-HPV) can promote the malignant transformation of HPV-infected cells through E6 and E7 viral oncoproteins, responsible for inactivating the *TP53* and *Rb* (retinoblastoma tumor suppressor gene) [7]. A subset of 12 alpha HR-HPV (16, 18, 31, 33, 35, 39, 45, 51, 52, 56, 58, and 59) has been classified as carcinogenic to humans according to the International Agency of Research in Cancer [8]. HR-HPV is considered the main cause of cervical cancer, genotypes 16 and 18 being responsible for 70% of cases [9]. In addition, several studies have also demonstrated the pathogenic role of HPV in other anogenital cancers [10–12] as well as in head and neck cancers [13]. Currently, HPV16 is widely recognized as an etiological factor in oropharynx tumors [14], however, not enough evidence exists regarding the HPV relationship and the anatomic subsites of head and neck squamous cell carcinoma [15].

Nowadays, a variety of molecular biological methods have been developed for the detection and genotyping of HPV at DNA, mRNA, and protein levels by polymerase chain reaction (PCR), real-time PCR, in situ hybridization, immunohistochemistry and serum antibody assays [16]. In addition, next-generation HPV sequencing approaches provide accurate information on genotype composition and pathways to better understand functional consequences [17]. Certain collection approaches present difficulties. For example, tumoral tissue biopsy is invasive and tumors may be inaccessible. For its part, the collection of oral exfoliated cells with cotton swabs or cytobrush is restricted to a specific and accessible oral area, making collection difficult for non-visual tumors and early molecular alterations. To overcome these drawbacks, the detection of HPV in oral exfoliated cells from saliva (with or without oral rinses) represents a quick and easy non-invasive alternative for oral and oropharyngeal cancer screening in high-risk populations. In this sense, several researchers have analyzed the prevalence of salivary HPV DNA from head and neck cancer, however, to our knowledge, no previous systematic review has elucidated evidence of this relationship. Therefore, the aim of the present systematic review and meta-analysis was to determine the prevalence and effect size of association between salivary HPV DNA and the risk of developing oral and oropharyngeal cancer.

2. Materials and Methods

2.1. Protocol and Registration

This study was conducted according to Preferred Reporting Items for Systematic Reviews and Meta-Analysis (PRISMA) guidelines [18] and the protocol was registered with the International Prospective Register of Systematic Reviews (reference No. CRD42020161345).

2.2. Search Strategy and Study Selection

The systematic literature search was performed in PubMed, EMBASE, Web of Science, LILACS, Scopus and the Cochrane Library through 9 January 2020, without language restrictions or specified start date. The following combinations of keywords and medical subject headings were used: (human papilloma virus OR HPV) AND (saliva OR oral rinses OR mouthwash) AND (oral squamous cell carcinoma OR OSCC OR oropharyngeal squamous cell carcinoma OR OPSCC OR oral cancer OR oropharyngeal cancer). All studies were screened based on the title and abstract, and eligible manuscripts were retrieved for full-text review. Additionally, we manually searched the reference lists in each original and review article in order to avoid missing potential studies. The literature search was performed independently by two researchers (ORG and MMSC), and any disagreements were resolved by consensus. The studies selected through the search strategy and other references were managed using RefWorks software, and duplicated items were removed using the associated tools.

2.3. Eligibility Criteria

We included the studies that met the following criteria: (1) case-control studies of patients with oral and/or oropharyngeal cancer and healthy controls, (2) HPV DNA prevalence determined in salivary samples (whole saliva or oral rinses), and (3) sufficient data to calculate odds ratios (ORs) with 95% confidence intervals (CIs). The exclusion criteria were as follows: (1) in vitro or animal study, (2) reviews, letters, personal opinions, book chapters, case reports, and conference abstracts, and (3) duplicate articles or suspicion of data overlap.

2.4. Protocol and Registration

Two researchers (ORG and MMSC) independently assessed each eligible manuscript, extracted data using a pre-established form, and collated the data into a Microsoft Excel spreadsheet (Microsoft Corp. Redmond, WA, USA). Any disagreement among reviewers was resolved by consensus. The following information was extracted from each study: author, publication year, country, type of sample, method of collection, tumor location, sample size, HPV detection method, number of cases and HPV-positive cases, number of controls and HPV-positive controls, HPV-positive genotypes, overall HPV DNA prevalence (number of subjects testing positive for any HPV type) and type-specific HPV DNA prevalence (number of subjects testing positive for specific HPV types: HPV16 or HPV18, HR-HPV and LR-HPV). If the required data were incomplete, attempts were made to contact the authors to obtain the missing information.

2.5. Assessment of Risk Bias

The Newcastle-Ottawa Scale (NOS) [19] was used to evaluate the individual quality of the selected studies by three independent researchers (ORG, ARF, and MMSC), and discrepancies were resolved by consensus. The NOS assesses the quality of non-randomized studies based on design, content and ease of use directed to the task of incorporating the quality assessments in the interpretation of meta-analytic results. This 'star system' consists of 8 items classified into three broad perspectives: the selection of study groups; the comparability of the groups; and the ascertainment of either the exposure or outcome of interest for case-control or cohort studies. The highest quality studies were allotted a maximum of one star for each item, except for, the item related to comparability, which was allowed the assignment of a maximum of two stars. The NOS score ranged from 0 to 9 stars and validity criteria were as follows: 8–9, high quality; 6–7, medium quality; <5 low quality.

2.6. Statistical Analysis

Statistical analysis was conducted using the meta package of free R software (v.3.5.2; https://www.r-project.org). Firstly, to evaluate the statistical model applied to the meta analytic database, heterogeneity was assessed using the Cochran's Q statistic test-based Chi-squared test and I2 statistics. Heterogeneity was considered significant when I2 > 50% and/or presence of a $p < 0.10$ for the Cochran's Q test. The prevalence of HPV DNA and HPV genotypes in oral and/or oropharyngeal cancer was calculated using fixed or random effects depending on the heterogeneity. The relationship between saliva HPV DNA infection and oral and/oropharyngeal cancer risk was evaluated by pooled odds ratio (OR) and 95% confidence intervals (CIs) comparing cases to controls. If significant heterogeneity was detected, the DerSimonian and Laird random-effects model was applied to calculate the pooled OR with 95% CIs; otherwise, the Mantel–Haenszel fixed-effects model was used. Then, subgroup analyses were performed to explore the potential sources of heterogeneity among studies according to the anatomic tumor location and HPV genotypes. Additionally, publication bias was checked with Begg's and Egger's tests and by visual inspection in funnel plots demonstrating the relationship between the individual log ORs and their standard errors [20,21]. *p*-values of <0.05 were considered to indicate statistical significance.

3. Results

3.1. Study Selection

A total of 1669 articles were identified across the six electronic databases and three additional reports from the reference lists. After removing duplicates, a total of 1542 articles were screened based on the title and abstract, and 1494 were excluded for lack of adherence to our inclusion criteria. Therefore, full-text articles were retrieved for the remaining 48 articles. After a full-text review, 34 articles were excluded for the following reasons: non case-control studies (22); controls under risk conditions (2); suspicious of data overlap (3); insufficient data (3); and reviews, letters, and meta-analysis (4). Finally, 14 articles met all the inclusion criteria and were included in the final analysis. A detailed flowchart showing the selection process is shown in Figure 1.

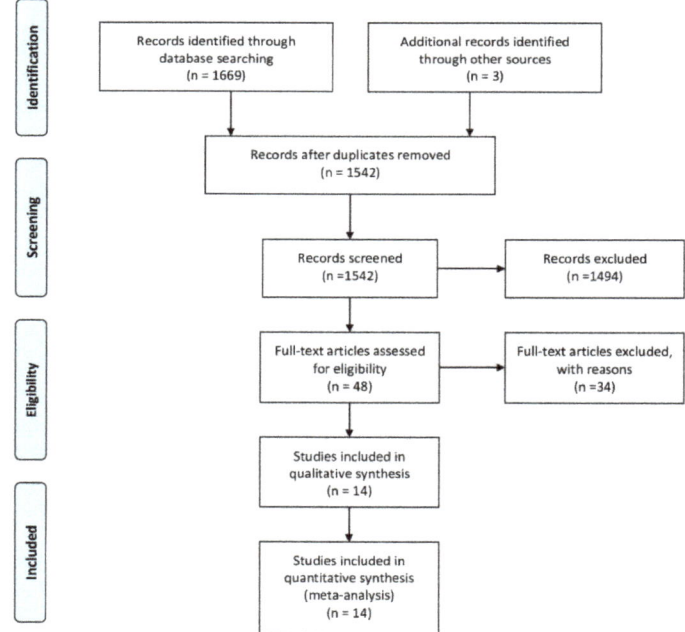

Figure 1. Preferred Reporting Items for Systematic Reviews and Meta-Analysis (PRISMA) flow diagram of the literature selection process, including identification, screening, eligibility and total studies included in qualitative and quantitative synthesis.

3.2. Study Characteristics

Individual characteristics of the included studies are summarized in Table 1. A total of 14 articles evaluating HPV prevalence in oral and/or oropharyngeal cancer were included in this meta-analysis, and these studies were carried out from 2005 to 2019. Study sample sizes ranged from 42 to 677 subjects.

The study units in this meta-analysis comprised a total of 2320 cases (658 from the oral cavity, 1160 from the oral cavity plus oropharynx and 502 from the oropharynx), and 5868 controls (2210 from the oral cavity, 2304 from the oral cavity plus oropharynx and 1354 from the oropharynx). As reported in Table 1, four studies were conducted in India [22–25], three in the USA [26–28], and two in Sweden [29,30], whereas the remaining studies were carried out in the following countries: Canada [31], France [32], Hungary [33], Pakistan [34], and Iran [35]. In terms of sampling, oral rinses and saliva ($n = 7$, 50%, respectively) were analyzed for HPV positivity and genotyping. The methods most used for saliva HPV-DNA determination were conventional PCR, nested PCR and quantitative PCR. However, other analytical strategies such as next generation sequencing or immunoassays were also employed for salivary HPV genotyping (Table 1).

3.3. Study Quality

Assessment of risk of bias and quality was performed according to NOS (Table S1). Regarding the selection domain, adequate description about characteristics and selection criteria for cases and controls were provided by all of the included studies. Regarding the comparability domain, six out of the 14 studies matched for age and at least one additional factor. Insofar as the exposure domain, few studies reported the blinding of analyses or non-response rates. The mean NOS score in our meta-analysis was six.

3.4. Meta-Analysis

3.4.1. Salivary HPV Association with Oral and Oropharyngeal Cancer

Overall, the prevalence of salivary HPV for oral and oropharyngeal carcinoma was of 43.2% ($n = 1160$) while the infection rate in the healthy control group was of 8.9% ($n = 2304$). Salivary HPV16 was the most common type of HPV DNA positive cases ($n = 1116$), representing 27.5% (Figure 2).

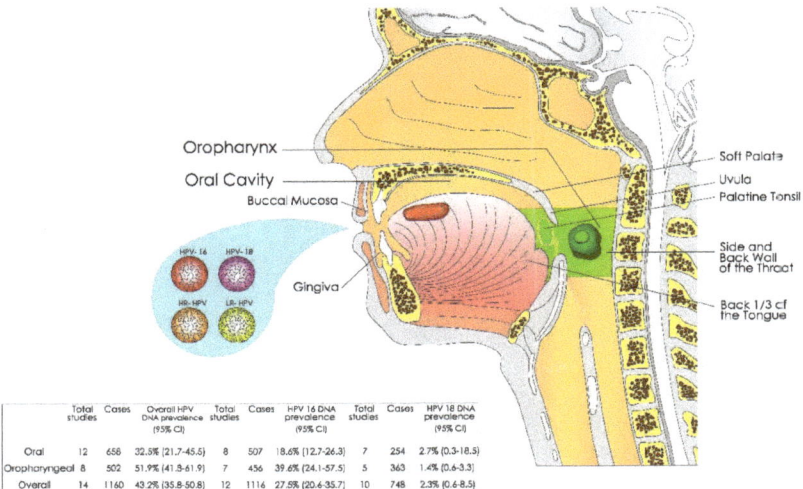

Figure 2. Schematic drawing of salivary HPV and prevalence of oral and/or oropharyngeal cancer. Oral tissue sheds pathogen-infected cells containing different HPV DNA genotypes (HPV16, HPV18, HR-HPV, and LR-HPV) into saliva (with or without oral rinses). The prevalence of salivary HPV DNA varied according to anatomic tumor location, showing the highest infection rate in oropharyngeal carcinomas. In addition, the type-specific prevalence in saliva was also different according to the anatomic tumor location.

Table 1. Characteristics of the 14 case-control studies included in this meta-analysis.

	Country	Tumor Location (n)	Type of Sample/ Method of Collection	HPV-Positive Cases (n/N)	HPV-Positive Case Types	HPV-Positive Controls (n/N)	HPV-Positive Control Types	HPV Detection Method
Hansson et al.; 2005	Sweden	OC (85) OPC (46)	Oral rinse/7 mL of 0.9% NaCl solution for 30s	39/131	16, 18, 33, 45, 58, 59, 13, 32, 62, 10, 76	14/320	16, 67, 54, 55, 62, 87, 75, 76, RTRX9	Nested PCR (MY09/ MY11 and GP5+/6+ primers) DNA sequencing
Saheblamee et al.; 2009	Iran	OC (22)	Oral rinse/10 mL of normal saline	9/22	16, 18, 6/11	5/20	16, 6/11	PCR (GP5+/6+ primers for L1 region)
Kulkarni et al.; 2011	India	OC (34)	Saliva	24/34	16, 18	255/396	16, 18	PCR (16 and 18 specific primers)
Goot-Heah et al.; 2012	India	OC (14)	Saliva	0/14	-	0/30	-	Nested PCR (MY09/11 and GP5+/6+ primers for L1 region)
Chen et al.; 2013	USA	OC (32) OPC (52)	Saliva/Oragene DNA kits (DNA Genotek)	38/84	16	1/19	16	qPCR (specific primers and probe for E6 region of HPV16)
Nordfors et al.; 2014	Sweden	OPC (47)	Oral rinse/15 mL 50% Listerine®/(Johnson and Johnson) for 30s	25/47	16, 18, 67, 6, 51	0/37	-	Bead-based multiplex assay on a MagPix instrument (Luminex Corporation), GP5+/6+ primers for the L1 region and specific primers and probe for E6 region of HPV16
Khyani et al.; 2015	Pakistan	OC (35)	Saliva	15/35	16, 18	3/35	16	qPCR using Real-time PCR Kit HPV16/18 Real-TM Quant (Sacace Biotechnologies)
Modak et al.; 2016	India	OC (235)	Saliva	149/235	16	193/409	16	PCR (HPV 16 specific primer)

Table 1. Cont.

Country	Tumor Location (n)	Type of Sample/Method of Collection	HPV-Positive Cases (n/N)	HPV-Positive Case Types	HPV-Positive Controls (n/N)	HPV-Positive Control Types	HPV Detection Method
Rosenthal et al.; 2017	USA	OC (61) OPC (45)	Oral rinse/10 mL of 0.9% NaCl solution for 30s	44/106	16, 18, * HR-HPV other	3/81	16, * HR-HPV other	qPCR from the HPV L1 region (Cobas®HPV Test-Roche Diagnostics)
Auguste et al.; 2017	France	OC (22) OPC (41)	Saliva/Oragene OG-500 kit (DNA Genotek)	21/63	16, 33, 51	80/308	16	PCR (SPF10 primer system for L1 region, INNO-LiPA®HPV Genotyping Extra; Innogenetics)
Laprise et al.; 2017	Canada	OC (72) OPC (183)	Oral rinse/alcohol-based solution for 15-30s	125/255	16, 18, ** HPV α-9 other than HPV16, *** HPV other	61/422	16, 18, ** HPV α-9 other than HPV16, *** HPV other	PCR (MY09/11 primers for HPV) and genotyping by Linear Array assay (Roche Molecular diagnostics)
Hettman et al.; 2018	Hungary	OPC (12)	Unstimulated saliva	4/12	16, 13	2/57	13, 11	PCR (MY09/11 primers for L1 region) Nested PCR (MY09/11 and GP5+/6+ primers for L1 region), sequencing for genotyping
Ramesh et al.; 2018	India	OC (30)	Oral rinse/10mL of 0.9% normal saline	13/30	16, 18	18/60	16, 18	Nested PCR (MY09/11 primers for L1 region)
Dang et al.; 2019	USA	OC (16) OPC (76)	Oral rinse/Original Mint Scope®mouthwash or Crest®Alcohol-free mouthwash (Proctor and Gamble) for 30s	37/92	16, NV14.4, NV69.1, NV95	1/110	18	qPCR (HPV16 E7/HPV18 E7 primers and probe) FAP-PCR from the L1 region NGS and Sanger sequencing

Abbreviations: OC, oral cancer; OPC, oropharynx cancer; PCR, polymerase chain reaction; qPCR, quantitative PCR; FAP-PCR, fluorescent arbitrarily primed PCR; NGS, next-generation sequencing; * HR-HPV other: 31, 33, 35, 39, 45, 51, 52, 56, 58, 59, 66, and 68; ** HPV α-9 other than HPV16: 31,33,35,52,58, and 67; *** HPV other: 6, 11, 18, 26, 34, 39, 40, 42, 44, 45, 51, 53, 54, 56, 59, 61, 62, 66, 68, 69, 70, 71, 72, 73, 81, 82, 83, 84, and 89.

Our meta-analysis included a total of 1160 cases and 2304 controls. The pooled analysis showed a significant association between positive salivary HPV DNA status and oral and oropharyngeal cancer with a pooled OR of 4.94 (95% CI = 2.82–8.67; $p < 0.01$) (Figure 3).

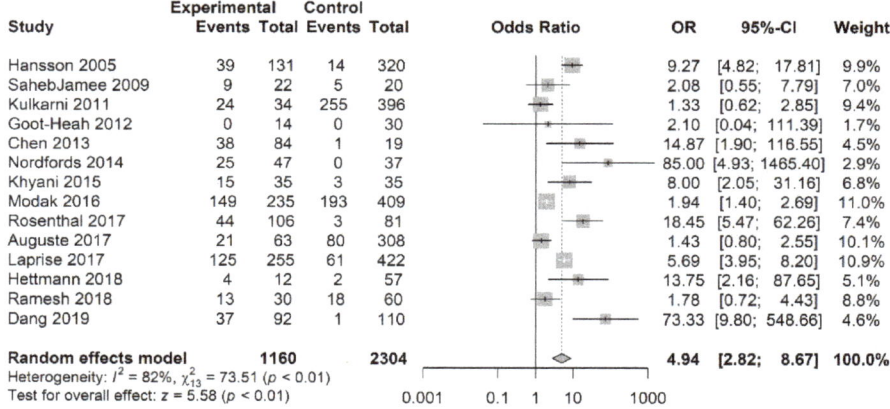

Figure 3. Forest plot for the studies on the association between salivary HPV and oral and oropharyngeal cancer. The squares indicate the ORs (odds ratios) in each study, with square sizes inversely proportional to the standard error of the OR. The diamond shape indicates the pooled ORs. Horizontal lines represent 95% CIs (confidence intervals), I2 > 50% indicates severe heterogeneity.

A random-effects model was used because heterogeneity was identified among the 14 studies (I2 = 82%). Visual inspection of the funnel plot revealed a symmetrical (Egger's test, $p = 0.159$; Begg's test, $p = 0.298$) distribution of the studies, indicating no evidence of publication bias (Figure 4).

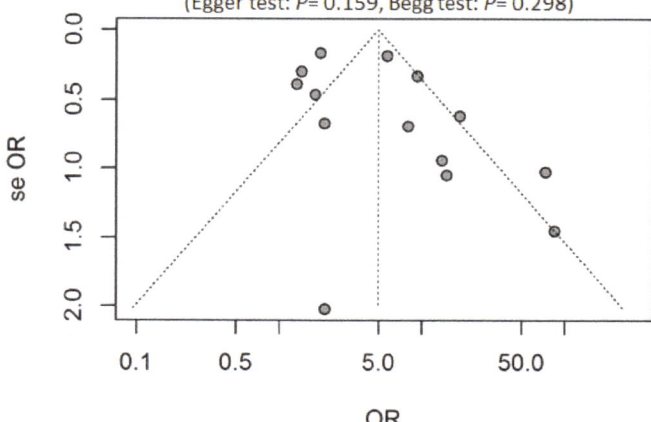

Figure 4. Funnel plot for studies (of 14 studies) on the association between salivary HPV and oral and oropharyngeal cancer. The vertical line represents the pooled OR using random-effect meta-analysis. Two diagonal lines represent (pseudo) 95% confidence limits around the OR for each standard error on the vertical axis. In the absence of heterogeneity, 95% of the studies should lie within the funnel defined by these diagonal lines. Abbreviations: se OR, standard error of odds ratio.

For the type-specific analysis (Figure 5), salivary HPV16 showed a significant association with a pooled OR of 10.07 (95% CI = 3.65–27.82; $p < 0.01$). However, salivary HPV18 did not show any significant increased risk for oral and oropharyngeal cancer with a pooled OR of 1.80 (95% CI = 0.66–4.90). In addition, a significant association was found for salivary HR-HPV with OR of 5.94 (95% CI = 2.78–12.69; $p < 0.01$), whereas salivary LR-HPV did not show any significant increased risk with OR of 1.45 (95% CI = 0.70–2.98). The respective funnel plots are represented in Figures S1–S4.

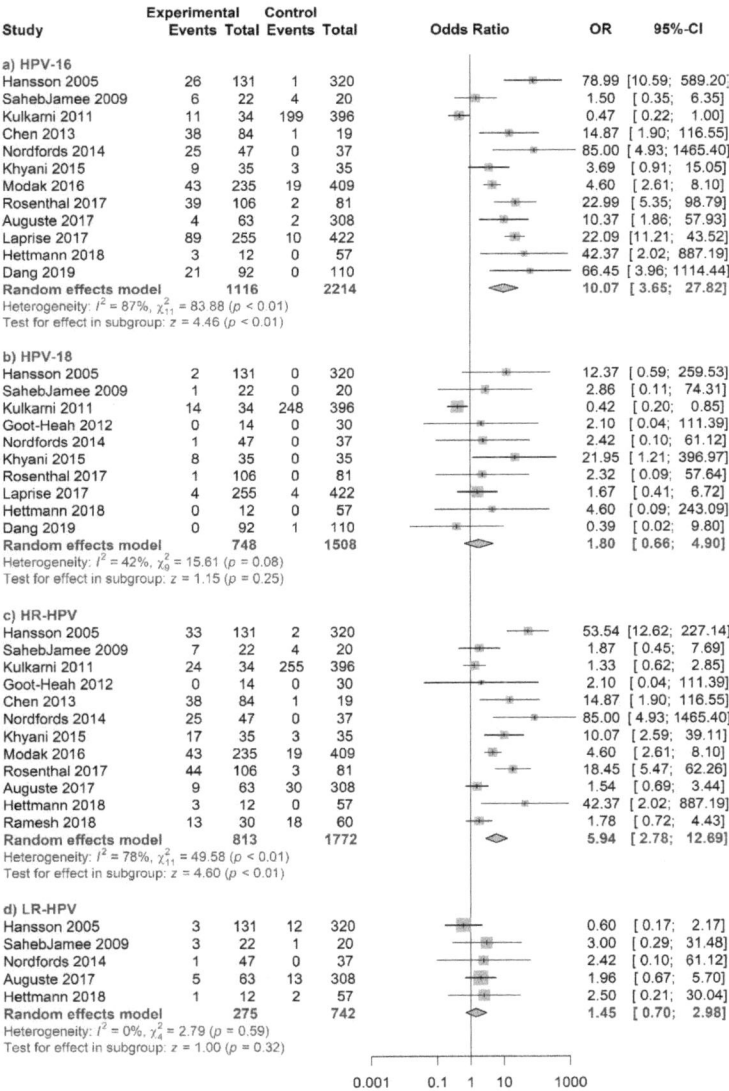

Figure 5. Forest plot for the studies on the association between salivary HPV and oral and oropharyngeal cancer. The squares indicate the ORs in each study, with square sizes inversely proportional to the standard error of the OR. The diamond shape indicates the pooled ORs. Horizontal lines represent 95% CIs. I2 > 50% indicates severe heterogeneity. (**a**) HPV16, (**b**) HPV18, (**c**) HR-HPV, and (**d**) LR-HPV.

3.4.2. Type-Specific Salivary HPV Association with Oropharyngeal Cancer

Our subgroup meta-analysis consisted of eight studies, including 502 cases and 1354 controls. In the pooled analysis, salivary HPV DNA infection and oropharyngeal cancer showed a significant association with a pooled OR of 17.71 (95% CI = 6.42–48.84; $p < 0.01$) (Figure 6).

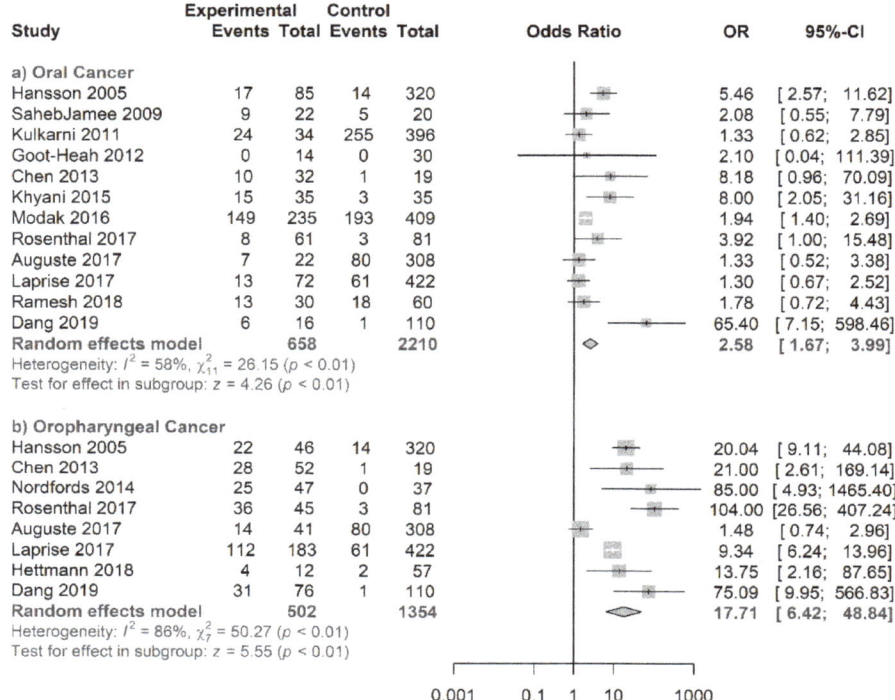

Figure 6. Forest plot for the studies on the association between salivary HPV and anatomic tumor subsites. The squares indicate the ORs in each study, with square sizes inversely proportional to the standard error of the OR. The diamond shape indicates the pooled ORs. Horizontal lines represent 95% CIs. I2 > 50% indicates severe heterogeneity. (**a**) Oral Cancer and (**b**) Oropharyngeal Cancer.

According to type-specific analysis (Figure 7), salivary HPV16 showed a significant association with a pooled OR of 38.50 (95% CI = 22.43–66.07; $p < 0.01$) whereas salivary HPV18 showed no significant association with a pooled OR of 1.92 (95% CI = 0.63–5.91). In addition, a significant association was found for salivary HR-HPV with a pooled OR of 26.69 (95% CI = 3.46–206.17; $p < 0.01$) whereas no significant association was found for salivary LR-HPV with a pooled OR of 2.08 (95% CI = 0.75–5.81). Their respective funnel plots are shown in Figures S5–S9.

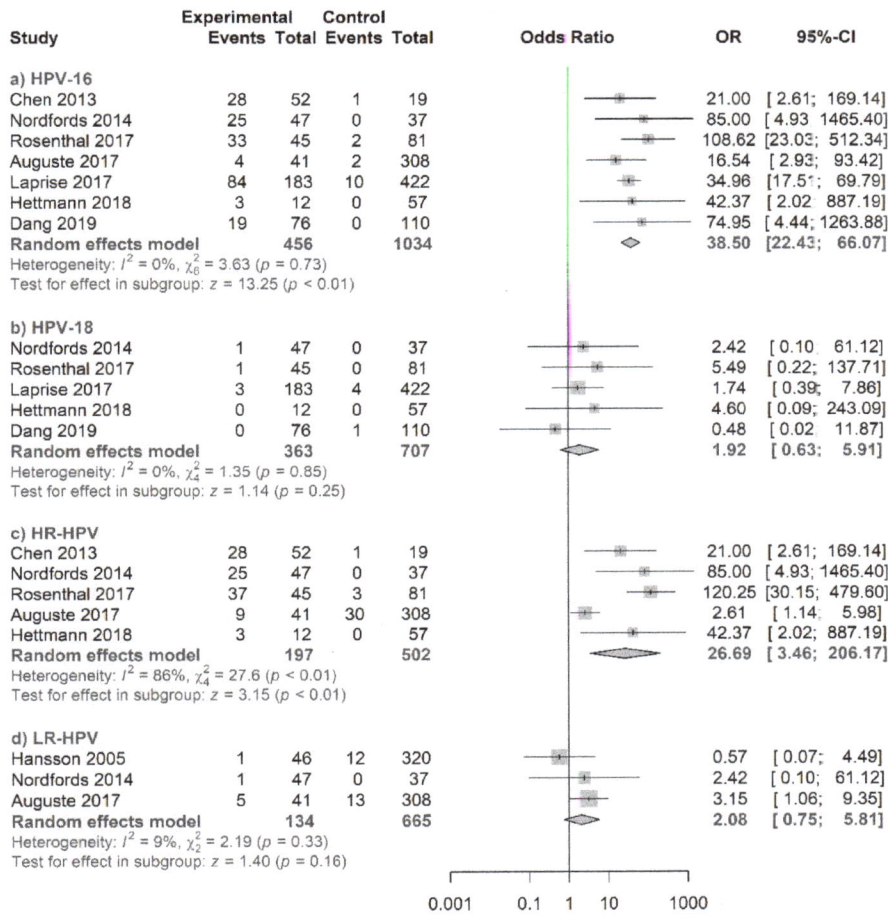

Figure 7. Forest plot for the studies on the association between salivary HPV and oropharyngeal cancer. The squares indicate the ORs in each study, with square sizes inversely proportional to the standard error of the OR. The diamond shape indicates the pooled ORs. Horizontal lines represent 95% CIs. I2 > 50% indicates severe heterogeneity. (**a**) HPV16, (**b**) HPV18, (**c**) HR-HPV, and (**d**) LR-HPV.

3.4.3. Type-Specific Salivary HPV Association with Oral Cancer

Our subgroup meta-analysis consisted of 12 studies, including 658 cases and 2210 controls. In the pooled analysis, salivary HPV DNA infection and oral cancer showed a significant association with a pooled OR of 2.58 (95% CI = 1.67–3.99; $p < 0.01$) (Figure 6). According to type-specific analysis (Figure 8), salivary HPV16 showed a significant association with a pooled OR of 2.95 (95% CI = 1.23–7.08; $p = 0.02$), whereas no significant association was observed for salivary HPV18 with a pooled OR of 1.51 (95% CI = 0.45–5.15). In addition, a significant association was observed for salivary HR-HPV with a pooled OR of 4.44 (95% CI = 2.47–7.98; $p < 0.01$). However, salivary LR-HPV did not show any significantly increased risk for oral cancer with OR of 1.79 (95% CI = 0.67–4.74). Their respective funnel plots are shown in Figures S10–S14.

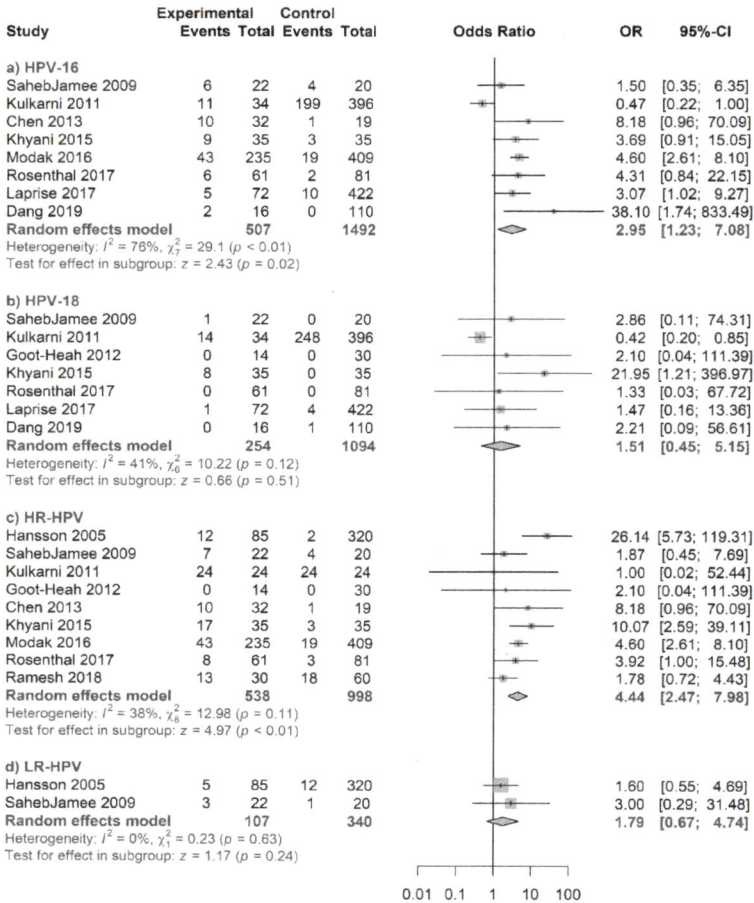

Figure 8. Forest plot for the studies on the association between salivary HPV and oral cancer. The squares indicate the ORs in each study, with square sizes inversely proportional to the standard error of the OR. The diamond shape indicates the pooled ORs. Horizontal lines represent 95% CIs. I2 > 50% indicates severe heterogeneity. (**a**) HPV16, (**b**) HPV18, (**c**) HR-HPV, and (**d**) LR-HPV.

4. Discussion

In the present study the overall pooled prevalence of salivary HPV-related to oral and oropharyngeal cancer was 43.2%. Similarly, a meta-analysis based on 11 case-control studies evaluating the HPV infection in oral and oropharyngeal cancer found an HPV DNA prevalence of 39.27% [36]. In terms of anatomic tumor location, we observed the highest prevalence of salivary HPV in oropharyngeal cancer (51.9%), whereas the overall percentage in the oral cavity was 32.5%. Similarly, a large comprehensive meta-analysis based on data from 148 studies estimated a pooled HPV DNA prevalence of 45.8% in oropharynx tumors and 24.5% in oral cavity tumors [37]. Although our meta-analysis did not evaluate HPV DNA prevalence in different oropharynx subsites, evidence shows that HPV is most prevalent in tonsils and base of tongue cancers compared to tumors located in walls of oropharynx, uvula and soft palate [38].

Overall, in our study, salivary HPV16 was the most commonly detected oncogenic type, accounting for around 28% of cases. As we expected, salivary HPV16 showed a higher prevalence in oropharyngeal cancer (39.6%) than oral cancer (18.6%), in accordance with previous studies [37,39,40]. In particular, the salivary HPV16 prevalence in our study was slightly higher in oral cancer than reported in a meta-analysis by Nydiae et al. [37] (18.6% vs 14.9%), however, other authors have reported higher rates of HPV16 prevalence in oral carcinoma, ranging from 20% to 50% [41–43]. Salivary HPV18 was another oncogenic HPV type commonly evaluated by the included studies. Unlike salivary HPV16, HPV18 positivity was found much less frequently, with an overall prevalence of 2.3%. Salivary HPV18 prevalence was even lower in oropharynx tumors (1.7%) as compared to oral cavity tumors (2.7%). One plausible explanation for the decreased prevalence of salivary HPV18 in both oral and oropharyngeal cancers is its specific tropism for glandular tissue and adenocarcinomas, while most head and neck cancers are predominantly of the squamous cell carcinoma type [44]. In addition, HR-HPV has developed a variety of mechanisms facilitating HPV evasion of recognition and clearance by the host immune system [45], which probably contributes to the different viral persistence in each of the anatomic regions of the head and neck. As in our study, Kreimer et al. [40] and Ndyae et al. [37] also found a low HPV18 prevalence in oropharynx tumors (1% and 0.7%, respectively), however, these studies reported a higher HPV18 prevalence in oral cancer (8% and 5.9%, respectively). These differences could be explained by the effect on HPV prevalence of different covariates such as geographical location, lifestyles (alcohol, tobacco or sexual activity), sample size, types of samples and methods used for HPV detection.

To the best of our knowledge, this is the first meta-analysis evaluating the association between salivary HPV and oral and/or oropharyngeal cancer. The pooled OR showed that oral and oropharyngeal cancer patients had an almost five-fold higher risk of HPV infection than controls. A previous meta-analysis evaluating the presence of HPV in oral and oropharyngeal cancer detected by different methods (histopathology, serum analysis, and cytopathology using OralCDx or oral swishes) reported a significant association with an OR of 2.82 [36]. Overall, our results indicate that salivary HPV causes a higher risk of oral and oropharyngeal carcinogenesis. In addition, we also conducted different subgroup analysis to evaluate the impact of HPV infection on cancer risk according to anatomic tumor location and HPV genotypes. We stratified the salivary HPV studies by anatomical location observing a stronger association between salivary HPV and oropharynx tumors compared to oral cavity tumors. Similarly, Shaik et al. performed a comprehensive metanalysis of HPV-associated head and neck cancers, reporting the highest association for oropharyngeal cancer, with an OR of 14.66, whereas oral cavity and laryngeal cancers had ORs of 4.06 and 3.23, respectively [46]. In addition, we evaluated type-specific salivary HPV risk associated with oral and oropharyngeal cancer. Compared to oncogenic potential, salivary HR-HPV types were associated with an increased risk of oral and oropharyngeal carcinomas. Thus, salivary HPV16 was significantly associated with oral cancer, confirming the findings reported in previous studies [43,47]. Like our study, Hobbs et al. reported a weak statistically significant association between HPV16 and oral cancer, with an OR of 2.0 [45]. On the contrary, a higher association (OR = 9) was reported by Zhu et al., suggesting the potential oncogenic role of HPV16 in oral carcinogenesis in Chinese population [43]. However, in our study, a stronger association was found between salivary HPV16 and oropharyngeal cancer, presenting an OR of 38.50, which suggests the role of HPV16 in the etiology of oropharyngeal cancer. Unlike other meta-analysis [47,48], our study did not analyze association based on specific subsites of the oropharynx. In this sense, a consistent association between HPV16 infection and tonsil cancer has previously been described [47], which seems to indicate a different oncogenic role for HPV infection in the different subsites of oropharynx.

All the studies included in the present meta-analysis addressed HPV status in oral exfoliated cells collected from saliva with or without oral rinses. In this sense, the first association between oral HPV and oral cancer was reported by Smith et al. [49]. These authors evaluated HPV status in oral exfoliated cells collected by oral rinses from 93 patients and 205 controls finding significantly increased risk (OR = 3.70) of cancer in positive oral HPV patients regardless of alcohol and tobacco use [49]. According to the evidence, salivary HPV DNA represents a promising approach for identifying oral HPV infection. Several authors have shown a significant correlation between HPV DNA detected in tissue and positivity for HPV DNA in saliva, suggesting the potential value of this biofluid for detecting HPV and thus predicting HPV-related head and neck carcinomas [1,50]. Furthermore, salivary HPV DNA has demonstrated to be a good marker for detecting HPV in oropharyngeal cancer, as a high agreement between salivary HPV16 DNA infection and tumor p16 expression has been observed [51–53]. However, a recent study revealed a lower sensitivity for identifying p16-positive oral cancer patients through salivary HPV, which may indicate a limited involvement of HPV16 in oral carcinogenesis [54]. Interestingly, our study reviewed the different salivary HPV genotypes identified in oral and oropharyngeal carcinomas, providing additional evidence on the co-existence of multiple HPV types during carcinogenesis. In this matter, saliva analysis represents a great opportunity for the identification and characterization of novel HPVs involved in head and neck cancer.

Our study has several strengths. It is the first meta-analysis highlighting the association between salivary HPV infection and oral and/or oropharyngeal cancer. Moreover, we examined both the overall and the specific prevalence of salivary HPV DNA in oral and/or oropharyngeal cancer. In addition, we performed a comprehensive literature review without language restrictions and the results of our study were in concordance with the scientific evidence. However, the present study is not exempt from limitations. Firstly, the studies included in our meta-analysis were heterogeneous, which could be explained by different factors such as ethnicity, sample size, geographic region, anatomic tumor location, method of HPV detection and different HPV genotypes. Although we performed a subgroup analysis by anatomic tumor location and HPV genotypes, we were unable to elucidate the potential sources contributing to this heterogeneity. Secondly, data such as age, smoking, drinking, sexual habits or diet were not provided by the studies in our sample, hampering the assessment of these confounding variables. Thirdly, some studies included in our analysis could be biased due to the fact that cases and controls were not matched for demographic variables such as age, sex and lifestyle habits. In addition, although almost all these studies analyzed HPV16 and HPV18, we observed high variability regarding HPV genotypes and HPV detection methods, which could substantially affect the results of our analysis.

5. Conclusions

To the best of our knowledge, this is the first meta-analysis addressing the association between salivary HPV infection and oral and oropharyngeal carcinoma. The findings of this meta-analysis provide additional evidence that salivary HPV is associated with oral and oropharyngeal cancer, suggesting that salivary HPV infection is a risk factor for oral and oropharyngeal cancer. However, to validate our findings, future research should focus on prospective cohort studies that explore the occurrence of salivary HPV infection in oral and oropharyngeal cancer. In addition, it is necessary to analyze confounding variables that might be associated with an increased risk of HPV infection in oral and oropharyngeal cancer.

Supplementary Materials: The following are available online at http://www.mdpi.com/2077-0383/9/5/1305/s1, Table S1: The Newcastle–Ottawa Scale (NOS) for assessing the quality of included studies, Figure S1: funnel plot for studies (of 12 studies) on the association between salivary HPV16 and oral and oropharyngeal cancer, Figure S2: funnel plot for studies (of 10 studies) on the association between salivary HPV18 and oral and oropharyngeal cancer, Figure S3: funnel plot for studies (of 12 studies) on the association between salivary HR-HPV and oral and oropharyngeal cancer, Figure S4: funnel plot for studies (of five studies) on the association between salivary LR-HPV and oral and oropharyngeal cancer, Figure S5: funnel plot for studies (of eight studies) on the association between salivary HPV and oropharyngeal cancer, Figure S6: funnel plot for studies (of seven studies) on the association between salivary HPV16 and oropharyngeal cancer, Figure S7: funnel plot for studies (of five studies) on the association between salivary HPV18 and oropharyngeal cancer, Figure S8: funnel plot for studies (of five studies) on the association between salivary HR-HPV and oropharyngeal cancer, Figure S9: funnel plot for studies (of three studies) on the association between salivary LR-HPV and oropharyngeal cancer, Figure S10: funnel plot for studies (of 12 studies) on the association between salivary HPV and oral cancer, Figure S11: funnel plot for studies (of eight studies) on the association between salivary HPV16 and oral cancer, Figure S12: funnel plot for studies (of seven studies) on the association between salivary HPV18 and oral cancer, Figure S13: funnel plot for studies (of nine studies) on the association between salivary HR-HPV and oral cancer, and Figure S14: funnel plot for studies (of two studies) on the association between salivary LR-HPV and oral cancer.

Author Contributions: Conceptualization, Ó.R.-G., R.L.-L. and M.M.S.-C.; methodology, Ó.R.-G., M.M.S.-C., Á.S.-B., and C.M.-R.; software, Á.S.-B. and C.M.-R.; validation, Ó.R.-G. and M.M.S.-C.; formal analysis, Á.S.-B. and C.M.-R.; investigation, Ó.R.-G. and M.M.S.-C.; resources, Ó.R.-G. and A.R.-F.; data curation, Á.S.-B. and C.M.-R.; writing—original draft preparation, Ó.R.-G. and M.M.S.-C.; writing—review and editing, Ó.R.-G. and M.M.S.-C., L.M.-R., R.L.-L., S.A.-L. and L.L.-M.; visualization, Ó.R.-G. and M.M.S.-C.; supervision, M.M.S.-C. and R.L.-L.; project administration, M.M.S.-C. and R.L.-L.; funding acquisition, M.M.S.-C. All authors have read and agreed to the published version of the manuscript.

Funding: This research received no external funding.

Conflicts of Interest: R.L.-L. reports other from Nasasbiotech, during the conduct of the study; grants and personal fees from Roche, grants and personal fees from Merck, personal fees from AstraZeneca, personal fees from Bayer, personal fees and non-financial support from BMS, personal fees from Pharmamar, personal fees from Leo, outside the submitted work. The rest of the authors have nothing to disclose.

References

1. Smith, E.M.; Ritchie, J.M.; Summersgill, K.F.; Hoffman, H.T.; Wang, D.H.; Haugen, T.H.; Turek, L.P. Human papillomavirus in oral exfoliated cells and risk of head and neck cancer. *J. Natl. Cancer Inst.* **2004**, *96*, 449–455. [CrossRef] [PubMed]
2. D'Souza, G.; Kreimer, A.R.; Viscidi, R.; Pawlita, M.; Fakhry, C.; Koch, W.M.; Westra, W.H.; Gillison, M.L. Case-control study of human papillomavirus and oropharyngeal cancer. *N. Engl. J. Med.* **2007**, *356*, 1944–1956. [CrossRef] [PubMed]
3. Murtaza, M.; Dawson, S.J.; Tsui, D.W.Y.; Gale, D.; Forshew, T.; Piskorz, A.M.; Parkinson, C.; Chin, S.F.; Kingsbury, Z.; Wong, A.S.C.; et al. Non-invasive analysis of acquired resistance to cancer therapy by sequencing of plasma DNA. *Nature* **2013**, *497*, 108–112. [CrossRef] [PubMed]
4. Fakhry, C.; Westra, W.H.; Li, S.; Cmelak, A.; Ridge, J.A.; Pinto, H.; Forastiere, A.; Gillison, M.L. Improved survival of patients with human papillomavirus-positive head and neck squamous cell carcinoma in a prospective clinical trial. *J. Natl. Cancer Inst.* **2008**, *100*, 261–269. [CrossRef]
5. O'Rorke, M.A.; Ellison, M.V.; Murray, L.J.; Moran, M.; James, J.; Anderson, L.A. Human papillomavirus related head and neck cancer survival: A systematic review and meta-analysis. *Oral Oncol.* **2012**, *48*, 1191–1201. [CrossRef]
6. Tommasino, M. The human papillomavirus family and its role in carcinogenesis. *Semin. Cancer Biol.* **2014**, *26*, 13–21. [CrossRef]
7. Sabatini, M.E.; Chiocca, S. Human papillomavirus as a driver of head and neck cancers. *Br. J. Cancer* **2020**, *122*, 306–314. [CrossRef]
8. IARC Working Group on the Evaluation of Carcinogenic Risks to Humans. Human papillomaviruses. *IARC Monogr. Eval. Carcinog. Risks Hum.* **2007**, *90*, 1–636.
9. Schiffman, M.; Castle, P.E.; Jeronimo, J.; Rodriguez, A.C.; Wacholder, S. Human papillomavirus and cervical cancer. *Lancet (Lond. Engl.)* **2007**, *370*, 890–907. [CrossRef]
10. Faber, M.T.; Sand, F.L.; Albieri, V.; Norrild, B.; Kjaer, S.K.; Verdoodt, F. Prevalence and type distribution of human papillomavirus in squamous cell carcinoma and intraepithelial neoplasia of the vulva. *Int. J. Cancer* **2017**, *141*, 1161–1169. [CrossRef]
11. Schlenker, B.; Schneede, P. The role of human papilloma virus in penile cancer prevention and new therapeutic agents. *Eur. Urol. Focus* **2019**, *5*, 42–45. [CrossRef] [PubMed]
12. Lin, C.; Franceschi, S.; Clifford, G.M. Human papillomavirus types from infection to cancer in the anus, according to sex and HIV status: A systematic review and meta-analysis. *Lancet Infect. Dis.* **2018**, *18*, 198–206. [CrossRef]
13. Tumban, E. A current update on human papillomavirus-associated head and neck cancers. *Viruses* **2019**, *11*, 922. [CrossRef] [PubMed]
14. IARC Working Group on the Evaluation of Carcinogenic Risks to Humans. Biological agents. Volume 100 B. A review of human carcinogens. *IARC Monogr. Eval. Carcinog. Risks Hum.* **2012**, *100 (Pt B)*, 1–441.
15. Hübbers, C.U.; Akgül, B. HPV and cancer of the oral cavity. *Virulence* **2015**, *6*, 244–248. [CrossRef]
16. Kobayashi, K.; Hisamatsu, K.; Suzui, N.; Hara, A.; Tomita, H.; Miyazaki, T. A review of HPV-related head and neck cancer. *J. Clin. Med.* **2018**, *7*, 241. [CrossRef]

17. Tuna, M.; Amos, C.I. Next generation sequencing and its applications in HPV-associated cancers. *Oncotarget* **2017**, *8*, 8877–8889. [CrossRef]
18. Moher, D.; Liberati, A.; Tetzlaff, J.; Altman, D.G. Preferred reporting items for systematic reviews and meta-analyses: The PRISMA Statement. *PLoS Med.* **2009**, *6*, e1000097. [CrossRef]
19. Wells, G.A.; Shea, B.; O'Connell, D.; Peterson, J.; Welch, V.; Losos, M.; Tugwell, P. The Newcastle-Ottawa Scale (NOS) for Assessing the Quality of Nonrandomized Studies in Meta-Analysis. Available online: http://www.ohri.ca/programs/clinical_epidemiology/oxford.asp (accessed on 18 February 2020).
20. Egger, M.; Davey Smith, G.; Schneider, M.; Minder, C. Bias in meta-analysis detected by a simple, graphical test. *BMJ* **1997**, *315*, 629–634. [CrossRef]
21. Begg, C.B.; Mazumdar, M. Operating characteristics of a rank correlation test for publication bias. *Biometrics* **1994**, *50*, 1088–1101. [CrossRef]
22. Kulkarni, S.S.; Kulkarni, S.S.; Vastrad, P.P.; Kulkarni, B.B.; Markande, A.R.; Kadakol, G.S.; Hiremath, S.V.; Kaliwal, S.; Patil, B.R.; Gai, P.B. Prevalence and distribution of high risk human papillomavirus (HPV) types 16 and 18 in carcinoma of cervix, saliva of patients with oral squamous cell carcinoma and in the general population in Karnataka, India. *Asian Pac. J. Cancer Prev.* **2011**, *12*, 645–648. [PubMed]
23. Goot-Heah, K.; Kwai-Lin, T.; Froemming, G.R.A.; Abraham, M.T.; Nik Mohd Rosdy, N.M.M.; Zain, R.B. Human papilloma virus 18 detection in oral squamous cell carcinoma and potentially malignant lesions using saliva samples. *Asian Pac. J. Cancer Prev.* **2012**, *13*, 6109–6113. [CrossRef]
24. Modak, H.; Sayad, T.; Fernandes, N. Molecular detection of HPV 16 in saliva of patients with oral squamous cell carcinoma and in the normal population of Southwesterly Indians. *Int. J. Adv. Biol. Res.* **2016**, *6*, 25–29.
25. Ramesh, P.S.; Devegowda, D.; Naik, P.R.; Doddamani, P.; Nataraj, S.M. Evaluating the feasibility of nested PCR as a screening tool to detect HPV infection in saliva of oral squamous cell carcinoma subjects. *J. Clin. Diagnostic Res.* **2018**, *12*, BC22–BC25. [CrossRef]
26. Rosenthal, M.; Huang, B.; Katabi, N.; Migliacci, J.; Bryant, R.; Kaplan, S.; Blackwell, T.; Patel, S.; Yang, L.; Pei, Z.; et al. Detection of HPV related oropharyngeal cancer in oral rinse specimens. *Oncotarget* **2017**, *8*, 109393–109401. [CrossRef]
27. Chen, K.M.; Stephen, J.K.; Ghanem, T.; Stachler, R.; Gardner, G.; Jones, L.; Schweitzer, V.P.; Hall, F.; Divine, G.; Worsham, M.J. Human papilloma virus prevalence in a multiethnic screening population. *Otolaryngol. Neck Surg.* **2013**, *148*, 436–442. [CrossRef]
28. Dang, J.; Bruce, G.A.; Zhang, Q.; Kiviat, N.B. Identification and characterization of novel human papillomaviruses in oral rinse samples from oral cavity and oropharyngeal cancer patients. *J. Oral Biosci.* **2019**, *61*, 190–194. [CrossRef]
29. Hansson, B.G.; Rosenquist, K.; Antonsson, A.; Wennerberg, J.; Schildt, E.-B.; Bladström, A.; Andersson, G. Strong association between infection with human papillomavirus and oral and oropharyngeal squamous cell carcinoma: A population-based case-control study in southern Sweden. *Acta Otolaryngol.* **2005**, *125*, 1337–1344. [CrossRef]
30. Nordfors, C.; Vlastos, A.; Du, J.; Ahrlund-Richter, A.; Tertipis, N.; Grün, N.; Romanitan, M.; Haeggblom, L.; Roosaar, A.; Dahllöf, G.; et al. Human papillomavirus prevalence is high in oral samples of patients with tonsillar and base of tongue cancer. *Oral Oncol.* **2014**, *50*, 491–497. [CrossRef]
31. Laprise, C.; Madathil, S.A.; Schlecht, N.F.; Castonguay, G.; Soulières, D.; Nguyen-Tan, P.F.; Allison, P.; Coutlée, F.; Hier, M.; Rousseau, M.C.; et al. Human papillomavirus genotypes and risk of head and neck cancers: Results from the HeNCe Life case-control study. *Oral Oncol.* **2017**, *69*, 56–61. [CrossRef]
32. Auguste, A.; Gaëte, S.; Herrmann-Storck, C.; Michineau, L.; Joachim, C.; Deloumeaux, J.; Duflo, S.; Luce, D. Prevalence of oral HPV infection among healthy individuals and head and neck cancer cases in the French West Indies. *Cancer Causes Control.* **2017**, *28*, 1333–1340. [CrossRef] [PubMed]
33. Hettmann, A.; Demcsák, A.; Bach, Á.; Decsi, G.; Dencs, Á.; Pálinkó, D.; Rovó, L.; Terhes, G.; Urbán, E.; Buzás, K.; et al. Prevalence and genotypes of human papillomavirus in saliva and tumor samples of head and neck cancer patients in Hungary. *Infect. Genet. Evol.* **2018**, *59*, 99–106. [CrossRef] [PubMed]
34. Khyani, I.A.M.; Qureshi, M.A.; Mirza, T.; Farooq, M.U. Salivary detection of human papilloma virus 16 & 18 in pre-malignant and malignant lesions of oral cavity: Is it feasible in Pakistani context of socio-cultural taboos? *Pak. J. Med. Sci.* **2015**, *31*, 1104–1109. [PubMed]

35. SahebJamee, M.; Boorghani, M.; Ghaffari, S.R.; AtarbashiMoghadam, F.; Keyhani, A. Human papillomavirus in saliva of patients with oral squamous cell carcinoma. *Med. Oral Patol. Oral Cir. Bucal* **2009**, *14*, e525–e528. [CrossRef]
36. Chaitanya, N.C.; Allam, N.S.; Gandhi Babu, D.B.; Waghray, S.; Badam, R.K.; Lavanya, R. Systematic meta-analysis on association of human papilloma virus and oral cancer. *J. Cancer Res. Ther.* **2016**, *12*, 969–974. [CrossRef]
37. Ndiaye, C.; Mena, M.; Alemany, L.; Arbyn, M.; Castellsagué, X.; Laporte, L.; Bosch, F.X.; de Sanjosé, S.; Trottier, H. HPV DNA, E6/E7 mRNA, and p16INK4a detection in head and neck cancers: A systematic review and meta-analysis. *Lancet Oncol.* **2014**, *15*, 1319–1331. [CrossRef]
38. Haeggblom, L.; Ramqvist, T.; Tommasino, M.; Dalianis, T.; Näsman, A. Time to change perspectives on HPV in oropharyngeal cancer. A systematic review of HPV prevalence per oropharyngeal sub-site the last 3 years. *Papillomavirus Res. (Amst. Neth.)* **2017**, *4*, 1–11. [CrossRef]
39. Guo, L.; Yang, F.; Yin, Y.; Liu, S.; Li, P.; Zhang, X.; Chen, D.; Liu, Y.; Wang, J.; Wang, K.; et al. Prevalence of human papillomavirus type-16 in head and neck cancer among the Chinese Population: A Meta-Analysis. *Front. Oncol.* **2018**, *8*, 619. [CrossRef]
40. Kreimer, A.R.; Clifford, G.M.; Boyle, P.; Franceschi, S. Human papillomavirus types in head and neck squamous cell carcinomas worldwide: A systematic review. *Cancer Epidemiol. Biomark. Prev.* **2005**, *14*, 467–475. [CrossRef]
41. Smitha, T.; Mohan, C.V.; Hemavathy, S. Prevalence of human papillomavirus16 DNA and p16INK4a protein in oral squamous cell carcinoma: A systematic review and meta-analysis. *J. Oral Maxillofac. Pathol.* **2017**, *21*, 76–81. [CrossRef]
42. Termine, N.; Panzarella, V.; Falaschini, S.; Russo, A.; Matranga, D.; Lo Muzio, L.; Campisi, G. HPV in oral squamous cell carcinoma vs head and neck squamous cell carcinoma biopsies: A meta-analysis (1988–2007). *Ann. Oncol.* **2008**, *19*, 1681–1690. [CrossRef] [PubMed]
43. Zhu, C.; Ling, Y.; Dong, C.; Zhou, X.; Wang, F. The relationship between oral squamous cell carcinoma and human papillomavirus: A meta-analysis of a Chinese population (1994–2011). *PLoS ONE* **2012**, *7*, e36294. [CrossRef]
44. Clifford, G.; Franceschi, S. Members of the human papillomavirus type 18 family (alpha-7 species) share a common association with adenocarcinoma of the cervix. *Int. J. Cancer* **2008**, *122*, 1684–1685. [CrossRef] [PubMed]
45. Grabowska, A.K.; Riemer, A.B. The invisible enemy—How human papillomaviruses avoid recognition and clearance by the host immune system. *Open Virol. J.* **2012**, *6*, 249–256. [CrossRef] [PubMed]
46. Shaikh, M.H.; McMillan, N.A.J.; Johnson, N.W. HPV-associated head and neck cancers in the Asia Pacific: A critical literature review & meta-analysis. *Cancer Epidemiol.* **2015**, *39*, 923–938. [PubMed]
47. Hobbs, C.G.L.; Sterne, J.A.C.; Bailey, M.; Heyderman, R.S.; Birchall, M.A.; Thomas, S.J. Human papillomavirus and head and neck cancer: A systematic review and meta-analysis. *Clin. Otolaryngol.* **2006**, *31*, 259–266. [CrossRef]
48. Saulle, R.; Semyonov, L.; Mannocci, A.; Careri, A.; Saburri, F.; Ottolenghi, L.; Guerra, F.; La Torre, G. Human papillomavirus and cancerous diseases of the head and neck: A systematic review and meta-analysis. *Oral Dis.* **2015**, *21*, 417–431. [CrossRef]
49. Smith, E.M.; Hoffman, H.T.; Summersgill, K.S.; Kirchner, H.L.; Turek, L.P.; Haugen, T.H. Human papillomavirus and risk of oral cancer. *Laryngoscope* **1998**, *108*, 1098–1103. [CrossRef]
50. Zhao, M.; Rosenbaum, E.; Carvalho, A.L.; Koch, W.; Jiang, W.; Sidransky, D.; Califano, J. Feasibility of quantitative PCR-based saliva rinse screening of HPV for head and neck cancer. *Int. J. Cancer* **2005**, *117*, 605–610. [CrossRef]
51. Chai, R.C.; Lim, Y.; Frazer, I.H.; Wan, Y.; Perry, C.; Jones, L.; Lambie, D.; Punyadeera, C. A pilot study to compare the detection of HPV-16 biomarkers in salivary oral rinses with tumour p16(INK4a) expression in head and neck squamous cell carcinoma patients. *BMC Cancer* **2016**, *16*, 178. [CrossRef]
52. Martin-Gomez, L.; Fulp, W.J.; Schell, M.J.; Sirak, B.; Abrahamsen, M.; Isaacs-Soriano, K.A.; Lorincz, A.; Wenig, B.; Chung, C.H.; Caudell, J.J.; et al. Oral gargle-tumor biopsy human papillomavirus (HPV) agreement and associated factors among oropharyngeal squamous cell carcinoma (OPSCC) cases. *Oral Oncol.* **2019**, *92*, 85–91. [CrossRef] [PubMed]

53. Tang, K.D.; Baeten, K.; Kenny, L.; Frazer, I.H.; Scheper, G.; Punyadeera, C. Unlocking the potential of saliva-based test to detect HPV-16-driven oropharyngeal cancer. *Cancers* **2019**, *11*, 473. [CrossRef] [PubMed]
54. Tang, K.D.; Menezes, L.; Baeten, K.; Walsh, L.J.; Whitfield, B.C.S.; Batstone, M.D.; Kenny, L.; Frazer, I.H.; Scheper, G.C.; Punyadeera, C. Oral HPV16 prevalence in oral potentially malignant disorders and oral cavity cancers. *Biomolecules* **2020**, *10*, 223. [CrossRef] [PubMed]

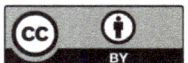

© 2020 by the authors. Licensee MDPI, Basel, Switzerland. This article is an open access article distributed under the terms and conditions of the Creative Commons Attribution (CC BY) license (http://creativecommons.org/licenses/by/4.0/).

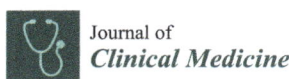

Review

Saliva and Oral Diseases

Emanuela Martina [†], Anna Campanati *,[†], Federico Diotallevi and Annamaria Offidani

Dermatology Clinic, Department of Clinical and Molecular Sciences, Polytechnic Marche University, via Conca 71, 60126 Ancona, Italy; ema.martina@gmail.com (E.M.); federico.diotallevi@hotmail.it (F.D.); a.offidani@ospedaliriuniti.marche.it (A.O.)
* Correspondence: anna.campanati@gmail.com; Tel.: +39-0715963433
† These authors contributed equally to the manuscript.

Received: 29 December 2019; Accepted: 3 February 2020; Published: 8 February 2020

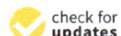

Abstract: Saliva is a fascinating biological fluid which has all the features of a perfect diagnostic tool. In fact, its collection is rapid, simple, and noninvasive. Thanks to several transport mechanisms and its intimate contact with crevicular fluid, saliva contains hundreds of proteins deriving from plasma. Advances in analytical techniques have opened a new era—called "salivaomics"—that investigates the salivary proteome, transcriptome, microRNAs, metabolome, and microbiome. In recent years, researchers have tried to find salivary biomarkers for oral and systemic diseases with various protocols and technologies. The review aspires to provide an overall perspective of salivary biomarkers concerning oral diseases such as lichen planus, oral cancer, blistering diseases, and psoriasis. Saliva has proved to be a promising substrate for the early detection of oral diseases and the evaluation of therapeutic response. However, the wide variation in sampling, processing, and measuring of salivary elements still represents a limit for the application in clinical practice.

Keywords: biomarkers; saliva; oral cancer; oral lichen planus; psoriasis; oral diseases

1. Introduction

Saliva is a biological fluid secreted by major and minor salivary glands. The major salivary glands are the parotid, submandibular, and sublingual glands. Minor salivary glands are widely disseminated throughout the entire oral cavity. Saliva provides lubrication; facilitates mastication, digestion, and taste; it has antimicrobial properties; and serves as buffer for acidic food. Moreover, saliva inhibits the demineralization of teeth and protects from caries [1]. The physiological secretion generates 0.75–1.5 L per day, with a decrease during the night [2]. Saliva contains 99% water and proteins for the remaining 1% (mucins, enzymes, immunoglobulins), electrolytes, lipids, and inorganic substances [3].

There are many advantages to employing saliva as a substrate for diagnostic analysis. Its sampling is fast, inexpensive, non-invasive, and well tolerated by children and people with disabilities; moreover, it is a safe procedure for healthcare providers [4]. Many serum substances enter saliva through passive diffusion, active transport, or extracellular ultrafiltration [5]. Obviously, compared with blood, levels of several analytes are lower, which was an obstacle until a few years ago [6]. Nowadays, highly sensitive molecular methods are available and can be used in the detection of many elements in saliva, despite their dimensions and concentrations [7].

In recent decades, enormous progress has been made in early diagnosis and screening for many diseases, especially for neoplastic conditions. However, some of these methods are invasive or expensive, and for certain conditions, accurate tests are still not available. This is the case for oral cancer, the sixth most common cancer worldwide, frequently diagnosed at an advanced stage with a 5 year survival rate of 50% [8].

In accordance with Biomarkers Definitions Working Group 2011, a biomarker is a characteristic that can be objectively measured and evaluated as indicator of normal biological or pathogenic processes, or as an indicator of pharmacologic response to therapeutic interventions [9]. The detection of salivary biomarkers and their use in clinical practice in the near future is one of the most ambitious aims of contemporary researchers.

2. Materials and Methods

The review was conducted in accordance with the PRISMA (Preferred Reporting Items for Systematic Reviews and Meta-Analyses) checklist. A search in the PubMed database was carried out using the keywords "saliva", "salivary", "biomarkers", "oral diseases", "oral lichen planus", "oral cancer", and associations between terms. We selected only articles written in English. The papers were selected first by analyzing titles and abstracts, in order to choose a correct match with our topic; full-text articles were then studied and included in the revision.

3. Sampling and Processing Techniques

Many factors can alter the composition and total amount of saliva. The time of day, hydration, body position, drugs intake, smoking, psychological stimuli, food assumption, and other factors related to systemic conditions can change the characteristics of saliva in a single subject [10]. A sample of saliva can be collected at rest or after stimulation. This procedure consists of offering a gum or swab to chew, or specific taste stimuli such as citric acid [11]. The stimulation changes not only the volume, but also the composition of saliva; it has been demonstrated that parasympathetic stimulation produces a high flow rate, but sympathetic stimulation produces a small flow richer in proteins and peptides [12]. Consequently, proteome profile and proportion are changeable as a reaction to neural activation [13].

As regards clinical trials, saliva is usually collected at rest ("unstimulated saliva") after at least 1 h of fasting, without drinking or smoking; the patient must be comfortably seated, avoid oro-facial movements for 5 min, and, just before the sampling, has to rinse their mouth with deionized water [11].

Saliva specimens can be collected from whole saliva or from a single gland (for example, the parotid gland). This procedure, which uses a different method, can be uncomfortable for patients and therefore is rarely used [14]. It should be specified that whole saliva has a higher proportion of non-salivary materials such as food debris, bacteria, desquamated epithelial cells, and leukocytes [15].

The gold standard method is to drain saliva using special devices (Salivette®, Sarstedt, Nümbrecht, Germany; Quantisal®, Immunalysis, Pomona, CA, USA; Orapette®, Trinity Biotech, Dublin, Ireland and SCS® Greiner Bio-One, Kremsmünster, Austria) [16].

Controversies are evident in the literature regarding centrifugation and speed, addition of PIC (protease inhibitor cocktail), and storage temperature. Most authors recommended the use of a protease inhibitor mixture in order to stabilize the substrate; moreover, the samples collected must be immediately stored in ice containers and, after processing, stored at −80 °C [17]. All these steps are necessary for bacterial growth inhibition and the minimal impairment of salivary proteins.

4. "Salivaomics"

The term "salivaomics" was coined in 2008 to emphasize the various "omics" found in saliva: genome, transcriptome, proteome, metabolome, and microbiome [18]. Salivaomics has been widely studied in recent years thanks to the advent of more advanced analytical techniques. Nearly 70% of the genome in saliva is human; the remaining 30% belongs to the oral microbiota [19]. The DNA contained in saliva is approximately 24 μg (range 0.2–52 μg), which is almost 10 times lower than in blood, but genotyping techniques require as little as 5 ng/mL of DNA to work effectively [20]. Polymerase chain reaction (PCR) and sequencing arrays can be applied to saliva samples. The analysis of salivary DNA aims especially to detect aberrant DNA methylation, which is the first epigenetic mark of neoplastic alterations [21].

4.1. Transcriptomes

mRNA and microRNA secreted from cells can be easily detected in saliva. Reverse transcriptase polymerase chain reaction and microarray are the most commonly used analyses. Zhang et al. first developed a technique to permit stabilization and to process salivary RNA [22]. The great potential of transcriptome study in the early detection of cancer and other diseases has been reported [23–25]. More recently, noncoding RNAs (ncRNAs) or microRNAs (miRNA) have been the subject of many studies because of their role in oncogenesis and their great stability in biological fluids, including saliva [26]. MicroRNAs are encoded by genes but are not translated into proteins; it is now generally accepted that these small nucleotides are involved in cell differentiation, proliferation, and survival. Moreover, many studies have already demonstrated the dysregulation of miRNAs in cancer tissues [27,28]. Surprisingly, salivary microRNAs are more stable than mRNAs, which makes this biological fluid a suitable substrate for transcriptome analysis.

4.2. Metabolome

The endogenous metabolites are nucleic acids, vitamins, lipids, organic acids, carbohydrates, thiols, and amino acids. The study of the salivary metabolome can provide an overview of the general health status or modification during systemic diseases [29]. In 2010, Sugimoto et al. first used salivary metabolome analysis with capillary electrophoresis and mass spectrometry to detect differences between healthy controls and patients with solid cancer [30]. The authors identified three metabolites that were oral-cancer-specific and eight metabolites that were pancreatic-cancer-specific. Nuclear magnetic resonance (NMR) spectroscopy can detect and measure metabolites in a solution with minimal sample preparation. This quantitative technique is based on the magnetic properties of atomic nuclei [31]. Each compound has a characteristic resonance frequency that makes it easy to distinguish. Moreover, the area under a signal peak is proportional to the concentration of the metabolite [32]. Liquid chromatography–mass spectrometry (LC-MS) is considered the gold standard in metabolomics. In fact, it is able to analyze an enormous range of analytes with a greater sensitivity than NMR [33]. This technique provides very high chromatographic resolution and its results are easily interpretable using libraries of molecular fragmentation patterns [34].

4.3. Proteome

The term "proteome" encompasses all proteins in the oral cavity. Saliva contains more than 2000 proteins with a multitude of biological activities [35] and one quarter of salivary proteins are detectable in plasma. The greatest obstacle to salivary proteome analysis is its rapid degradation, which occurs just minutes after sample collection. For this reason, the majority of researchers combine the saliva with protease inhibitor cocktails (PIC) before storage and analysis, as suggested by Xiao et al. [36]. Proteomics takes advantage of NMR spectroscopy and gas and liquid chromatography–mass spectrometry (GC-MS and LC-MS), described above. In this research field, two-dimensional polyacrylamide gel electrophoresis (2D-PAGE) and capillary electrophoresis with electrochemical detection are essential tools [37]. 2D-PAGE, which precedes the advent of 2D-difference gel electrophoresis (2D-DIGE), fractionates proteins on the basis of their isoelectric points in the first dimension and apparent molecular weight in the second [38]. An amphoteric carrier or an ampholyte is added to a gel and subjected to electrophoresis under a continuously regulated temperature. The acrylamide gel is placed in a glass tube and proteins are separated via an isoelectric gradient; it is easy to understand why this method is poorly accurate with multiple samples. 2D-DIGE dramatically improved 2D-PAGE thanks to the possibility of labeling each sample with distinct fluorescent dyes and then reading them using a laser scanner. Immunoassay is one of the most commonly used analytical techniques to detect the expression of an antibody or an antigen in a test sample. Enzyme-linked immunosorbent assay (ELISA) has been used for a variety of applications including diagnostic tools and quality controls [39]. The four basic setups are direct, indirect, sandwich, and competitive ELISAs. Direct ELISA is the simplest format, requiring an antigen and an enzyme-conjugated antibody specific to the antigen [40]. The ELISA method is a sensitive and specific test that rapidly produces results and for these advantages has found a wide field of applications in clinical practice (e.g., in viral serology tests).

4.4. Microbiome

The study of microbiota has probably been the largest topic in scientific literature in recent years. In fact, next-generation sequencing has allowed the identification of thousands of phylotypes of microorganism throughout the entire human body, and research is ongoing. About 19,000 microorganisms have been identified in saliva [41]. Oral dysbiosis can lead to periodontal disease [42], caries [43], and some evidence exists supporting an association with cancer and systemic diseases [44,45]. Nowadays, molecular biology methods such as 16S ribosomal RNA (rRNA) gene sequencing, polymerase chain reaction (PCR), and other related PCR-based methods are very popular thanks to their high sensitivity and reproducibility. However, these techniques are no longer employed in routine diagnostics due to their costs. Alternative approaches include electromigration techniques (two-dimensional gel electrophoresis, capillary zone electrophoresis) and MS methods, such as matrix-assisted laser desorption ionization time-of-flight mode (MALDI-TOF MS). MALDI-TOF MS is a fast and accurate method based on the ionization of intact microorganism cells with short laser pulses and the subsequent acceleration of the particles in a vacuum by way of an electric field. Each microorganism has a specific spectrum profile [46].

Histopathology, in some cases with direct immunofluorescence, remains the gold standard for the diagnosis of oral disease. In fact, it is often necessary to perform a biopsy to confirm the diagnosis of bullous diseases (together with DIF) [47], Sjögren's syndrome [48], and for all lesions suspected for malignancy [49].

5. Fields of Application

In this article, we have summarized the latest findings on the use of saliva as a diagnostic tool in oral inflammatory diseases. In particular, we chose the most epidemiologically relevant conditions or where the oral cavity is a typical location of a systemic disease. In fact, mouth disorders can often precede the onset of systemic symptoms (e.g., in bullous pemphigus), and early diagnosis of oral disease can change the prognosis of these patients. In this scenario, the study of salivary biomarkers is a promising tool for early diagnosis and screening in susceptible populations (e.g., in smokers).

5.1. Oral Lichen Planus

Oral lichen planus (OLP) is one of the most common chronic inflammatory condition of the oral mucosa, with 0.5%–2% prevalence in adults and a slight predominance in women [50]. OLP affects oral mucosa symmetrically, with a predilection for oral mucosa. Clinically, it is possible to distinguish different aspects: reticular (the most prevalent form), erythematous, ulcerative or erosive, plaque-like, bullous, or papular [51,52]. The histopathology of OLP is typical, with a prominent lymphocyte infiltrate at the interface of epithelium, acanthosis, and degeneration of the basal cell layer [53]. Direct immunofluorescence (DIF) permits deposition of Immunoglobulin M as colloid bodies and C3 in granular and linear patterns in the basement membrane zone to be detected [54]. Although the exact pathogenesis of OLP is mostly unknown, it is believed that autoreactive T cells play a crucial role in the disease. Several risks/triggers factors have been described, such as stress, HCV and viral infections, and drugs [55]. OLP has been classified as a premalignant lesion for its risk of malignant transformation (0.04–1.74 per year) in squamous cell carcinoma (OSCC) [56]. Patients affected by OLP suffer from burning and itching sensations up to a severe pain in the erosive form; the disease has a huge negative impact on quality of life due to impairment in daily activities such as eating or oral hygiene [57]. Published articles focused on salivary biomarkers in OLP are quite recent and concern the diagnosis of OLP, but in particular the early detection of malignant transformation.

In 2018, Sineepat et al. enrolled five OLP patients and five healthy controls using a proteomic approach on saliva with two-dimensional gel electrophoresis followed by mass spectrometry. The authors detected three proteins that showed a potential role in OLP patients (cystatin SA, chain C of human complement component C3c, and chain B of fibrinogen fragment D) and tested with ELISA. All the analytical techniques confirmed with statistical significance that fibrinogen fragment D and complement component C3c were increased and cystatin SA was decreased in OLP patients compared with healthy subjects [58]. Fibrinogen fragments D and C3c play a central role in inflammation, whereas cystatin SA belongs to the cystatin superfamily, a group of cysteine protease inhibitors with antimicrobial activity. In fact, fibrinogen expression and C3 deposition are typical findings in OLP using IFD [54].

A different and more complex panel of proteins was reported by another study, published in 2017 [59]. The study was conducted on 10 patients, investigating with mass spectrometry 108 proteins differentially expressed in OLP subjects in comparison to healthy controls. The first finding was the absence of proteins essential to lubrication and viscoelasticity, supporting the xerostomia symptom frequently reported by patients. The authors interestingly tried to link protein expression in saliva with histological findings in OLP, discussing the known functions of each peptide. In particular, S100A8 and S100A9 (also called MRP8 and MRP14) are calcium- and zinc-binding proteins with a role in inflammation and cytokine production via IL-17. S100A8 can also induce apoptosis via attraction to skin of $CD8^+$ cells and natural killer (NK) cells [60]. Another player in the scene of T-cell proliferation and differentiation is AZGP1 (zinc-alpha-2-glycoprotein), which is an adipocytokine [61]. The study also confirmed the crucial role of oxidative stress in OLP; reactive oxygen species (ROS) induce apoptosis and dysfunction in keratinocytes and, moreover, ROS can be further produced from $TCD4^+$ lymphocytes infiltrating in OLP in a vicious circle.

Oxidative stress in OLP was previously discussed in 2016 in a case–control study enrolling 62 patients and 30 healthy individuals [62]. The authors demonstrated significant differences between patients and the control group concerning the average concentration of total antioxidant capacity (TAC, determined using the Benzie and Strain method [26]), glutathione (GSH, measured spectrophotometrically), and thiobarbituric-acid-reactive substances (TBARS, determined using the Aust method), which are a product of lipid peroxidation [63]. In patients suffering from OLP, as expected, TAC and GSH had lower values, while TBARS was higher than in healthy controls. More interestingly, patients with an erosive form of lichen had more marked values, demonstrating severe oxidative stress and a great concordance with clinical features. These findings could support the oral or topical use of antioxidants [64].

Many authors have suggested salivary cortisol as a biomarker in OLP [65–70]. Cortisol is considered a biological marker of stress and anxiety, the variation of which can alter cytokine profiles [71]. OLP has a double connection with stress: anxiety and stressful events are considered a trigger for OLP onset but, at the same time, oral lichen itself represent a source of stress for patients. In this intricate scenario, the evaluation of salivary cortisol seems to mimic the ancestral question "Which came first, the chicken or the egg?" In fact, data from the literature are controversial, and cortisol is probably not suitable as a biomarker in OLP. As previously discussed, OLP is a T-cell-driven disease; however, it is still unclear if the inflammation is due to Th1 or Th2 expression. In fact, in OLP, there are numerous cytokines expressed both from recruited lymphocytes and from affected keratinocytes, in a mechanism of self-amplification [72]. The evaluation of specific interleukin in saliva is certainly a good trace to detect biomarkers in OLP and, moreover, to design tailored therapies. Nowadays, more consistent results concern IL-6 and IL-8. Interleukin-6 is involved in B- and T-cell differentiation and is able to inactivate p53 with tumor progression of some cancers [73]. Mozaffari et al. revealed in a meta-analysis that IL-6 levels in saliva and serum of OLP patients were significantly higher than in healthy controls, with higher values in saliva than in serum [74]. For this reason, saliva seemed to be more useful than serum for the detection of IL-6. Interleukin-8 is an important mediator of host response to injury and inflammation; it can activate neutrophils, basophils, and T cells [75]. The group of Mozaffari conducted a meta-analysis on this topic [76]. The most interesting finding was that IL-8 plays a key role in the transformation from reticular to erosive form of lichen, probably due to the loss of efficacy in the repairing mechanisms of keratinocytes [77]. IL-8 also revealed a potential application in therapeutic monitoring, as demonstrated via its decrease in saliva after dexamethasone administration [78].

5.2. Oral Cancer

Oral cancer is the sixth most common cancer worldwide [79] with a higher incidence in India, because of the chewing of areca nut/betel quid [80]. The mortality rate after 5 years from diagnosis is still 50% [79]. Well-known risk factors include tobacco consumption, alcohol abuse, and human papilloma virus infections [81]. The onset of an oral cancer is frequently asymptomatic, but most oral carcinomas develop from premalignant conditions such as leukoplakia and oral lichen planus [82,83]. Nowadays, the gold standard for diagnosis is tissue biopsy, an invasive technique that requires specific training and creates public health costs [84]. It is therefore easy to understand the need for an early detection method for pre-cancer and cancer by validating salivary biomarkers. Above, we discussed the great diagnostic potential of miRNA both in saliva and serum. In 2018, a well-designed study enrolled 30 patients with OLP, 15 patients with OSCC and 15 healthy donors [85]. Saliva samples were analyzed by quantitative RT-PCR for miR-21, miR-125a, miR31, and miR200a. Results showed that miRNA-21 and -125a were, respectively, higher and lower in OSCC patients and in OLP with dysplasia compared to healthy controls with statistical significance. miR-21 has been widely studied in oral, head, and neck cancer and has been postulated that it might have a role in inhibition of tumor suppression and apoptosis [86]. In contrast, miR-125a may act as a tumor suppressor, downregulating target oncogens [87]. Based on these data, the authors suggested a negative prognostic role of decreased salivary miR-125a levels in association with increased salivary miR-21 levels in OLP patients. Ishikawa et al. recently suggested a metabolomics approach to distinguish OLP from OSCC [88]; the authors detected higher levels of 12 salivary metabolites in OSCC patients compared with OLP patients. More specifically, the combination of indole-3-acetate and ethanolamine phosphate showed the best statistical accuracy. The aim of Mikkonen's research was to investigate the potential of nuclear magnetic resonance (NMR) spectroscopy for detecting the salivary metabolic changes associated with head and neck squamous cell carcinoma (HNSCC). The Authors found two metabolites, fucose and 1,2-propanediol, to be significantly upregulated, whereas proline was significantly downregulated in patients affected by HNSCC. The combination of four salivary metabolites (fucose, glycine, methanol, and proline) together provided maximum discrimination among HNSCC patients and healthy controls [31]. The role of fucosylation of glycoproteins in the development of cancer has been studied in recent years [89]. Ample evidence exists to prove that in normal tissues, fucosylation levels are relatively low, but this rapidly increases during carcinogenesis [90]. Aberrant glycosylation in cancer development is also an investigation area in oral diseases; in particular, researchers have focused attention on sialic acid (N-acetyl neuraminic acid), which is an important terminal sugar in cell membrane glycoproteins and glycolipids. Previous studies have shown elevated levels of salivary sialic acid in various carcinomas, including oral pre-cancer and OC [91–93].

The fascinating study of the microbiome has a wide field of application in the oral cavity. An extensive work has just been published regarding the alterations of salivary microbial community in oropharyngeal and hypopharyngeal carcinoma patients. In fact, the microbiome is considered a potential modulator of cancer metabolism [94]. The authors found 13 phylotypes of microorganism as potential diagnostic biomarkers in oral cancer. The role of the microbiome in malignant change in the oral cavity is still controversial because of the lack of large cohort studies. Healy et al. considered the implication of risk factors such as smoking or alcohol consumption in promoting epithelial dysplasia and production of carcinogenic agents [95]. Acetaldehyde (ACH) and N-nitrosamine compounds are potential genotoxic agents that are increased in the saliva of smokers; these compounds can be produced in vitro by microbial cultures [96,97]. In vitro studies have demonstrated the leading role of *Neisseria* species and *Candida* species in ACH production [98,99]. However, one study revealed the reduction of *Neisseria* species in the oral cavity of smokers, with a theoretical improvement of ACH levels [100]. Current theories hypothesize that the presence of these organisms could accelerate the progression of dysplasia towards OSCC in association with predisposing factors such as diet, age, or smoking/alcohol consumption habits in a multifactorial vision.

5.3. Blistering Diseases

Bullous pemphigoid (BP) and pemphigus vulgaris (PV) are acquired bullous diseases affecting the mucosa and/or skin. In both diseases, autoantibodies react with adhesion cell mechanisms or with the basement layer, resulting in blistering. Blisters are intraepithelial/intraepidermal in PV, whereas in BP they are subepithelial/subepidermal [101]. The diagnosis is first clinical, then confirmed with histopathology and direct immunofluorescence (IFD). In BP, bullae involving the skin and oral lesions are rare; in contrast, PV frequently begins with oral blistering or oral lesions following cutaneous involvement. IFD reveals IgG and C3 (BP180) deposition on the basement membrane in BP, while in PV it shows intercellular IgG antibody deposition to desmoglein (Dsg) 1 and/or desmoglein 3, which are trans-membrane desmosomal proteins [102]. In recent years, the use of ELISA to detect autoantibodies in the serum of BP and PV patients has entered clinical practice for diagnosis and therapeutic monitoring [101]. Starting from this technique, some authors have proposed the use of saliva as substrate for the research of BP180 and Dsg1 and 3. In 2006, Andreadis et al. first applied ELISA in both the serum and saliva of PV and BP patients, finding a great concordance in serum and saliva levels of Dsg1 and 3, while the BP180 determination on saliva failed [103]. Similar results emerged from Ali's study [104] on Dsg1 and 3. The potential of salivary testing in PV prognosis and mucosal severity has been investigated in two studies. Hallaji et al. included 50 patients with histologically confirmed PV and performed ELISA for Dsg1 and 3 on serum and saliva samples [105]. There was statistically significant concordance between serum and salivary levels of Dsg; more interestingly, there was a significant relationship between salivary anti-Dsg1 antibody and mucosal severity. The authors explained these data with the loss of integrity in mucosa and the largest transition of antibodies in saliva. The study of De et al. perfectly reproduced this finding and the authors perfectly agreed with the explanation concerning higher Dsg1 levels in severe disease [106]. In contrast to the previously discussed research, one Italian study was designed to assess the use of a BIOCHIP approach compared with ELISA in PV [107]. In fact, the authors considered saliva an unsuitable substrate for autoantibody detection because of the discordance between techniques found when using saliva samples.

5.4. Sjögren's Syndrome

Sjögren's syndrome (SS) is a systemic autoimmune disease characterized by the inflammation and consecutive destruction of exocrine glands, as well as salivary and lacrimal glands, with the occurrence of a lymphoepithelial sialadenitis [108]. The majority of patients are women of menopausal age; oral manifestations are frequently present at the onset of disease, but some patients develop a systemic disease with the involvement of joints, the gastrointestinal tract, the central nervous system, and with an increased risk of lymphoma [109]. Patients suffering from SS typically complain about xerostomia and its impact on their quality of life [110]. Current research on salivary biomarkers in SS is pursuing a non-invasive diagnostic test, a therapeutic monitoring marker, and, moreover, an early detection of lymphoma onset. One of the current diagnostic approaches is the detection of anti-Ro/SSA and/or anti-La/SSB in serum; studies from different groups have demonstrated the presence of these autoantibodies in the saliva of SS patients [111,112]. The determination of salivary autoantibodies seemed to be effective in discriminating SS patients from patients affected by systemic lupus erythematosus (SLE) [113]. A few studies have investigated cytokine profiles in SS saliva; data from these studies showed significantly higher levels of Th1, Th2, and Th17, in accordance with serum findings [114,115]. The proteomic approach in SS comprises proteins, enzymes, calcium-binding proteins, and immune-related molecules. Summarizing, data from the literature report high levels of inflammatory-phase proteins in saliva that can provide a great indication of gland status [116]. Lee et al.

recently published the results of determination of soluble sialic-acid-binding immunoglobulin-like lectin (siglec)-5 in saliva and sera by ELISA [117]. The level of salivary siglec-5 was significantly higher in the saliva from SS patients, which reflects the severity of hyposalivation. Several novel miRNAs have been described in SS [118]. Pauley et al. demonstrated that the expression of miR-146a was significantly increased in SS patients [119]. In Alevizos' research, another two miRNAs, miR-768-3p and miR-574, were associated with minor salivary gland inflammation in 15 patients with SS [120]. The pathogenesis of autoimmune diseases is a very complex interaction of many factors; epigenetic modifications are now considered crucial to the control of gene expression associated with these diseases [121,122]. Thabet et al. proposed that the dysfunction of salivary gland epithelial cells in SS might be partially linked to epigenetic modifications. Their analysis showed that blood global DNA methylation was reduced in SS patients and the expression of the gene DNMT1, which encodes DNA methyltransferase 1, was decreased compared to healthy controls. In contrast, the expression of the gene Gadd45a, which encodes the growth arrest and DNA-damage-inducible protein GADD45 alpha (GADD45a), was increased [123]. Probably the most interesting field in saliva and SS is the early diagnosis and prevention of MALT-type lymphoma [124]. The neoplasm has an insidious onset, almost asymptomatic, with a fast progression and dissemination. Cui et al. described a triad of markers (anti-cofillin-1, anti-alpha-enolase, and anti-Rho GDP-dissociation inhibitor 2) overexpressed in patients with SS who developed MALT lymphoma compared with SS patients and healthy individuals [125]. Sharma et al. recently examined the role of the microbiome in SS compared to healthy controls [126]. The analysis, performed with DNA isolation and 16rRNA sequencing, revealed four genera (Bifidobacterium, Dialister, Lactobacillus, and Leptotrichia) that were different between the two groups. The results were consistent with previous studies, revealing a role of Actinobacteria and Firmicutes phila [127,128]. More interestingly, Sharma et al. identified a difference in alpha diversity in patients treated with steroids, suggesting the potential role of microbiome analysis in therapeutic response.

5.5. Psoriasis

Psoriasis is now classified as an immune-mediated inflammatory disease (IMID) of the skin. It is being recognized that patients with psoriasis are at higher risk of developing systemic co-morbidities, e.g., metabolic syndrome and cardiovascular diseases [129,130].

Oral involvement in course of psoriasis is still debated. Recently, it has been hypothesized that gingivitis and periodontitis share the same underlying inflammatory pathogenic process as psoriasis. Thus, in our previous study, psoriatic patients were investigated for oral mucosa lesion prevalence as well as gum disease. Results displayed an increased association between gingivitis/periodontitis and psoriasis, which may suggest common underlying pathogenic risk factors [131].

Furthermore, salivary secretions, collected from patients with active psoriasis and healthy control subjects, were investigated for expression of interleukin (IL)-1b, IL-6, transforming growth factor (TGF)-β1, IL-8, tumor necrosis factor (TNF)-α, interferon (IFN)-χ, IL-17A, IL-4, IL-10, monocyte chemoattractant protein (MCP)-1, microphage inflammatory protein (MIP)-1a, and MIP-1b using a Multi-Analyte ELISArray Kit (Qiagen, Venlo, the Netherlands). Patients with active psoriasis had significantly higher salivary IL1β, TNF-α, TGF-β, and MCP-1 levels than healthy controls [132].

Thus, saliva can be a valid non-invasive tool for monitoring inflammation in psoriasis [133].

6. Conclusions

In the era of precision medicine, salivaomics approaches seem to be a promising field of research. Despite encouraging results reported in this review, there is a large variability in study designs, protocols, sampling collections, and techniques. Moreover, the study of new molecules with new technologies requires a well-established range of values without random decisions. Future studies should standardize accurate methodologies in order to validate new salivary biomarkers in clinical practice.

Author Contributions: E.M. was responsible for the literature revision and drafting; A.C. was responsible for final drafting and revision; F.D. contributed to article analysis; A.O. gave her final revision. All authors have read and agree to the published version of the manuscript.

Funding: This research received no external funding.

Conflicts of Interest: The authors declare no conflict of interest to declare.

References

1. Qin, R.; Steel, A.; Fazel, N. Oral mucosa biology and salivary biomarkers. *Clin. Dermatol.* **2017**, *35*, 477–483. [CrossRef] [PubMed]
2. Holmberg, K.V.; Hoffman, M.P. Anatomy, Biogenesis and Regeneration in Salivary Glands. *Monogr. Oral Sci.* **2014**, *24*, 1–13. [PubMed]
3. Mese, H.; Matsuo, R. Salivary secretion, taste and hyposalivation. *J. Oral Rehabil.* **2007**, *34*, 711–723. [CrossRef] [PubMed]
4. Kaczor-Urbanowicz, K.E.; Martin Carreras-Presas, C.; Aro, K.; Tu, M.; Garcia-Godoy, F.; Wong, D.T.W. Saliva diagnostics—Current views and directions. *Exp. Biol. Med.* **2017**, *242*, 459–472. [CrossRef]
5. Pfaffe, T.; Cooper-White, J.; Beyerlein, P.; Kostner, K.; Punyadeera, C. Diagnostic potential of saliva: Current state and future applications. *Clin. Chem.* **2011**, *57*, 675–687. [CrossRef]
6. Javaid, M.A.; Ahmed, A.S.; Durand, R.; Tran, S.D. Saliva as a diagnostic tool for oral and systemic diseases. *J. Oral Biol. Craniofacial Res.* **2016**, *6*, 67–76. [CrossRef]
7. Iguiniz, M.; Heinisch, S. Two-dimensional liquid chromatography in pharmaceutical analysis. Instrumental aspects, trends and applications. *J. Pharm. Biomed. Anal.* **2017**, *145*, 482–503. [CrossRef]
8. Petti, S. Pooled estimate of world leukoplakia prevalence: A systematic review. *Oral Oncol.* **2003**, *39*, 770–780. [CrossRef]
9. Delli, K.; Villa, A.; Farah, C.S.; Celentano, A.; Ojeda, D.; Peterson, D.; Jensen, S.B.; Glurich, I.; Vissink, A. World Workshop on Oral Medicine VII: Biomarkers predicting lymphoma in the salivary glands of patients with Sjögren's syndrome—A systematic review. *Oral Dis.* **2019**, *25*, 49–63. [CrossRef]
10. Siqueira, W.L.; Dawes, C. The salivary proteome: Challenges and perspectives. *PROTEOMICS Clin. Appl.* **2011**, *5*, 575–579. [CrossRef]
11. Navazesh, M. Methods for Collecting Saliva. *Ann. N. Y. Acad. Sci.* **1993**, *694*, 72–77. [CrossRef] [PubMed]
12. Lorenzo-Pouso, A.I.; Pérez-Sayáns, M.; Bravo, S.B.; López-Jornet, P.; García-Vence, M.; Alonso-Sampedro, M.; Carballo, J.; García-García, A.; Zalewska, A. Protein-Based Salivary Profiles as Novel Biomarkers for Oral Diseases. *Dis. Markers* **2018**, *2018*, 6141845. [CrossRef] [PubMed]
13. Proctor, G.B.; Carpenter, G.H. Salivary Secretion: Mechanism and Neural Regulation. In *Monographs in Oral Science*; KARGER: Basel, Switzerland, 2014; Volume 24, pp. 14–29. ISBN 0077-0892.
14. Henson, B.S.; Wong, D.T. Collection, Storage, and Processing of Saliva Samples for Downstream Molecular Applications. In *Oral Biology. Methods in Molecular Biology (Methods and Protocols)*; Humana Press: Totowa, NJ, USA, 2010; Volume 666H.
15. Kaufman, E.; Lamster, I.B. The diagnostic applications of saliva—A review. *Crit. Rev. Oral Biol. Med.* **2002**, *13*, 197–212. [CrossRef] [PubMed]
16. Khurshid, Z.; Zohaib, S.; Najeeb, S.; Zafar, M.S.; Slowey, P.D.; Almas, K. Human Saliva Collection Devices for Proteomics: An Update. *Int. J. Mol. Sci.* **2016**, *17*, 846. [CrossRef]
17. Schipper, R.; Loof, A.; de Groot, J.; Harthoorn, L.; Dransfield, E.; van Heerde, W. SELDI-TOF-MS of saliva: Methodology and pre-treatment effects. *J. Chromatogr. B* **2007**, *847*, 45–53. [CrossRef]
18. Ai, J.; Smith, B.; Wong, D.T. Saliva Ontology: An ontology-based framework for a Salivaomics Knowledge Base. *BMC Bioinform.* **2010**, *11*, 302. [CrossRef]
19. Rylander-Rudqvist, T.; Håkansson, N.; Tybring, G.; Wolk, A. Quality and Quantity of Saliva DNA Obtained from the Self-administrated Oragene Method—A Pilot Study on the Cohort of Swedish Men. *Cancer Epidemiol. Biomark. Prev.* **2006**, *15*, 1742–1745. [CrossRef]
20. Abraham, J.E.; Maranian, M.J.; Spiteri, I.; Russell, R.; Ingle, S.; Luccarini, C.; Earl, H.M.; Pharoah, P.P.D.; Dunning, A.M.; Caldas, C. Saliva samples are a viable alternative to blood samples as a source of DNA for high throughput genotyping. *BMC Med. Genom.* **2012**, *5*, 19. [CrossRef]

21. Gaździcka, J.; Gołąbek, K.; Strzelczyk, J.K.; Ostrowska, Z. Epigenetic Modifications in Head and Neck Cancer. *Biochem. Genet.* **2019**. [CrossRef]
22. Lee, Y.-H.; Zhou, H.; Reiss, J.K.; Yan, X.; Zhang, L.; Chia, D.; Wong, D.T.W. Direct Saliva Transcriptome Analysis. *Clin. Chem.* **2011**, *57*, 1295–1302. [CrossRef]
23. Tutar, Y. Editorial (Thematic Issue: "miRNA and Cancer; Computational and Experimental Approaches"). *Curr. Pharm. Biotechnol.* **2014**, *15*, 429. [CrossRef] [PubMed]
24. Kaczor-Urbanowicz, K.E.; Martín Carreras-Presas, C.; Kaczor, T.; Tu, M.; Wei, F.; Garcia-Godoy, F.; Wong, D.T.W. Emerging technologies for salivaomics in cancer detection. *J. Cell. Mol. Med.* **2017**, *21*, 640–647. [CrossRef] [PubMed]
25. Prattichizzo, F.; Giuliani, A.; Recchioni, R.; Bonafè, M.; Marcheselli, F.; De Carolis, S.; Campanati, A.; Giuliodori, K.; Rippo, M.R.; Brugè, F.; et al. Anti-TNF-α treatment modulates SASP and SASP-related microRNAs in endothelial cells and in circulating angiogenic cells. *Oncotarget* **2016**, *7*, 11945–11958. [CrossRef] [PubMed]
26. Majem, B.; Rigau, M.; Reventós, J.; Wong, D.T. Non-coding RNAs in saliva: Emerging biomarkers for molecular diagnostics. *Int. J. Mol. Sci.* **2015**, *16*, 8676–8698. [CrossRef]
27. Bartel, D.P. MicroRNAs: Target recognition and regulatory functions. *Cell* **2009**, *136*, 215–233. [CrossRef]
28. Adams, B.D.; Kasinski, A.L.; Slack, F.J. Aberrant regulation and function of microRNAs in cancer. *Curr. Biol.* **2014**, *24*, R762–R776. [CrossRef]
29. Bessonneau, V.; Bojko, B.; Pawliszyn, J. Analysis of human saliva metabolome by direct immersion solid-phase microextraction LC and benchtop orbitrap MS. *Bioanalysis* **2013**, *5*, 783–792. [CrossRef]
30. Sugimoto, M.; Wong, D.T.; Hirayama, A.; Soga, T.; Tomita, M. Capillary electrophoresis mass spectrometry-based saliva metabolomics identified oral, breast and pancreatic cancer-specific profiles. *Metabolomics* **2010**, *6*, 78–95. [CrossRef]
31. Mikkonen, J.J.W.; Singh, S.P.; Akhi, R.; Salo, T.; Lappalainen, R.; González-Arriagada, W.A.; Lopes, M.A.; Kullaa, A.M.; Myllymaa, S. Potential role of nuclear magnetic resonance spectroscopy to identify salivary metabolite alterations in patients with head and neck cancer. *Oncol. Lett.* **2018**, *16*, 6795–6800. [CrossRef]
32. Emwas, A.-H.M. The Strengths and Weaknesses of NMR Spectroscopy and Mass Spectrometry with Particular Focus on Metabolomics Research. In *Metabonomics: Methods and Protocols*; Bjerrum, J.T., Ed.; Springer: New York, NY, USA, 2015; pp. 161–193. ISBN 978-1-4939-2377-9.
33. McBride, E.M.; Lawrence, R.J.; McGee, K.; Mach, P.M.; Demond, P.S.; Busch, M.W.; Ramsay, J.W.; Hussey, E.K.; Glaros, T.; Dhummakupt, E.S. Rapid liquid chromatography tandem mass spectrometry method for targeted quantitation of human performance metabolites in saliva. *J. Chromatogr. A* **2019**, *1601*, 205–213. [CrossRef]
34. Beale, D.J.; Jones, O.A.H.; Karpe, A.V.; Dayalan, S.; Oh, D.Y.; Kouremenos, K.A.; Ahmed, W.; Palombo, E.A. A review of analytical techniques and their application in disease diagnosis in breathomics and salivaomics research. *Int. J. Mol. Sci.* **2017**, *18*, 24. [CrossRef] [PubMed]
35. Esteves, C.V.; de Campos, W.G.; de Souza, M.M.; Lourenço, S.V.; Siqueira, W.L.; Lemos-Júnior, C.A. Diagnostic potential of saliva proteome analysis: A review and guide to clinical practice. *Braz. Oral Res.* **2019**, *33*. [CrossRef] [PubMed]
36. Xiao, H.; Wong, D.T.W. Method development for proteome stabilization in human saliva. *Anal. Chim. Acta* **2012**, *722*, 63–69. [CrossRef] [PubMed]
37. Mishra, S.; Saadat, D.; Kwon, O.; Lee, Y.; Choi, W.S.; Kim, J.H.; Yeo, W.H. Recent advances in salivary cancer diagnostics enabled by biosensors and bioelectronics. *Biosens. Bioelectron.* **2016**, *81*, 181–197. [CrossRef]
38. Kondo, T. Cancer biomarker development and two-dimensional difference gel electrophoresis (2D-DIGE). *Biochim. Biophys. Acta Proteins Proteom.* **2019**, *1867*, 2–8. [CrossRef]
39. Zhang, Y.; Li, X.; Di, Y.P. Fast and Efficient Measurement of Clinical and Biological Samples Using Immunoassay-Based Multiplexing Systems. In *Molecular Toxicology Protocols*; Keohavong, P., Singh, K.P., Gao, W., Eds.; Springer: New York, NY, USA, 2020; pp. 129–147. ISBN 978-1-0716-0223-2.
40. Lin, A. V Direct ELISA. In *ELISA: Methods and Protocols*; Hnasko, R., Ed.; Springer: New York, NY, USA, 2015; pp. 61–67. ISBN 978-1-4939-2742-5.
41. Zaura, E.; Brandt, B.W.; Prodan, A.; Teixeira de Mattos, M.J.; Imangaliyev, S.; Kool, J.; Buijs, M.J.; Jagers, F.L.; Hennequin-Hoenderdos, N.L.; Slot, D.E.; et al. On the ecosystemic network of saliva in healthy young adults. *ISME J.* **2017**, *11*, 1218–1231. [CrossRef]

42. Ge, X.; Rodriguez, R.; Trinh, M.; Gunsolley, J.; Xu, P. Oral microbiome of deep and shallow dental pockets in chronic periodontitis. *PLoS ONE* **2013**, *8*, e65520. [CrossRef]
43. Burne, R.A.; Zeng, L.; Ahn, S.J.; Palmer, S.R.; Liu, Y.; Lefebure, T.; Stanhope, M.J.; Nascimento, M.M. Progress dissecting the oral microbiome in caries and health. *Adv. Dent. Res.* **2012**, *24*, 77–80. [CrossRef]
44. Schwabe, R.F.; Jobin, C. The microbiome and cancer. *Nat. Rev. Cancer* **2013**, *13*, 800–812. [CrossRef]
45. Torres, P.J.; Fletcher, E.M.; Gibbons, S.M.; Bouvet, M.; Doran, K.S.; Kelley, S.T. Characterization of the salivary microbiome in patients with pancreatic cancer. *PeerJ* **2015**, *3*, e1373. [CrossRef]
46. Buszewski, B.; Rogowska, A.; Pomastowski, P.; Złoch, M.; Railean-Plugaru, V. Identification of microorganisms by modern analytical techniques. *J. AOAC Int.* **2017**, *100*, 1607–1623. [CrossRef]
47. Rashid, H.; Lamberts, A.; Diercks, G.F.H.; Pas, H.H.; Meijer, J.M.; Bolling, M.C.; Horváth, B. Oral Lesions in Autoimmune Bullous Diseases: An Overview of Clinical Characteristics and Diagnostic Algorithm. *Am. J. Clin. Dermatol.* **2019**, *20*, 847–861. [CrossRef] [PubMed]
48. Jonsson, R.; Brokstad, K.A.; Jonsson, M.V.; Delaleu, N.; Skarstein, K. Current concepts on Sjögren's syndrome–classification criteria and biomarkers. *Eur. J. Oral Sci.* **2018**, *126*, 37–48. [CrossRef] [PubMed]
49. Warnakulasuriya, S. Oral potentially malignant disorders: A comprehensive review on clinical aspects and management. *Oral Oncol.* **2020**, *102*, 104550. [CrossRef] [PubMed]
50. McCartan, B.E.; Healy, C.M. The reported prevalence of oral lichen planus: A review and critique. *J. Oral Pathol. Med.* **2008**, *37*, 447–453. [CrossRef] [PubMed]
51. Thorn, J.J.; Holmstrup, P.; Rindum, J.P.J. Course of various clinical forms of oral lichen planus. A prospective follow-up study of 611 patients. *J. Oral Pathol.* **1988**, *17*, 213–218. [CrossRef] [PubMed]
52. Campanati, A.; Brandozzi, G.; Giangiacomi, M.; Simonetti, O.; Marconi, B.; Offidani, A.M. Lichen striatus in adults and pimecrolimus: Open, off-label clinical study. *Int. J. Dermatol.* **2008**, *47*, 732–736. [CrossRef]
53. Cheng, Y.-S.L.; Gould, A.; Kurago, Z.; Fantasia, J.; Muller, S. Diagnosis of oral lichen planus: A position paper of the American Academy of Oral and Maxillofacial Pathology. *Oral Surg. Oral Med. Oral Pathol. Oral Radiol.* **2016**, *122*, 332–354. [CrossRef]
54. Buajeeb, W.; Okuma, N.; Thanakun, S.; Laothumthut, T. Direct Immunofluorescence in Oral Lichen Planus. *J. Clin. Diagn. Res.* **2015**, *9*, ZC34–ZC37. [CrossRef]
55. Lodi, G.; Scully, C.; Carrozzo, M.; Griffiths, M.; Sugerman, P.B.; Thongprasom, K. Current controversies in oral lichen planus: Report of an international consensus meeting. Part 1. Viral infections and etiopathogenesis. *Oral Surg. Oral Med. Oral Pathol. Oral Radiol.* **2005**, *100*, 40–51. [CrossRef]
56. Van der Meij, E.H.; Schepman, K.-P.; van der Waal, I. The possible premalignant character of oral lichen planus and oral lichenoid lesions: A prospective study. *Oral Surg. Oral Med. Oral Pathol. Oral Radiol.* **2003**, *96*, 164–171. [CrossRef]
57. Radwan-Oczko, M.; Zwyrtek, E.; Owczarek, J.E.; Szcześniak, D. Psychopathological profile and quality of life of patients with oral lichen planus. *J. Appl. Oral Sci.* **2018**, *26*, e20170146. [CrossRef] [PubMed]
58. Talungchit, S.; Buajeeb, W.; Lerdtripop, C.; Surarit, R.; Chairatvit, K.; Roytrakul, S.; Kobayashi, H.; Izumi, Y.; Khovidhunkit, S.-o.P. Putative salivary protein biomarkers for the diagnosis of oral lichen planus: A case-control study. *BMC Oral Health* **2018**, *18*, 42. [CrossRef] [PubMed]
59. Souza, M.M.; Florezi, G.P.; Nico, M.M.S.; de Paula, F.; Paula, F.M.; Lourenço, S.V. Salivary proteomics in lichen planus: A relationship with pathogenesis? *Oral Dis.* **2018**, *24*, 784–792. [CrossRef]
60. De Carvalho, G.C.; Domingues, R.; de Sousa Nogueira, M.A.; Branco, A.C.C.; Manfrere, K.C.G.; Pereira, N.V.; Aoki, V.; Sotto, M.N.; da Silva Duarte, A.J.; Sato, M.N. Up-regulation of Proinflammatory Genes and Cytokines Induced by S100A8 in CD8 + T Cells in Lichen Planus. *Acta Derm. Venereol.* **2016**, *96*, 485–489. [CrossRef]
61. Severo, J.S.; Morais, J.B.S.; Beserra, J.B.; dos Santos, L.R.; de Sousa Melo, S.R.; de Sousa, G.S.; de Matos Neto, E.M.; Henriques, G.S.; do Nascimento Marreiro, D. Role of Zinc in Zinc-α2-Glycoprotein Metabolism in Obesity: A Review of Literature. *Biol. Trace Elem. Res.* **2020**, *193*, 81–88. [CrossRef]
62. Darczuk, D.; Krzysciak, W.; Vyhouskaya, P.; Kesek, B.; Galecka-Wanatowicz, D.; Lipska, W.; Kaczmarzyk, T.; Gluch-Lutwin, K.; Mordyl, B.; Chomyszyn-Gajewska, M. Salivary oxidative status in patients with oral lichen planus. *J. Physiol. Pharmacol.* **2016**, *67*, 885–894.
63. Abdolsamadi, H.; Rafieian, N.; Goodarzi, M.T.; Feradmal, J.; Davoodi, P.; Jazayeri, M.; Taghavi, Z.; Hoseyni, S.-H.; Ahmadi-Motamayel, F. Levels of salivary antioxidant vitamins and lipid peroxidation in patients with oral lichen planus and healthy individuals. *Chonnam Med. J.* **2014**, *50*, 58–62. [CrossRef]

64. Rivarola de Gutierrez, E.; Di Fabio, A.; Salomón, S.; Lanfranchi, H. Topical treatment of oral lichen planus with anthocyanins. *Med. Oral Patol. Oral Cir. Bucal* **2014**, *19*, e459–e466. [CrossRef]
65. Skrinjar, I.; Vidranski, V.; Brzak, B.L.; Juras, D.V.; Rogulj, A.A.; Brailo, V.; Boras, V.V. Salivary cortisol levels in patients with oral lichen planus—A pilot case-control study. *Dent. J.* **2019**, *7*, 59. [CrossRef]
66. Mansourian, A.; Najafi, S.; Nojoumi, N.; Parhami, P.M.M. Salivary Cortisol and Salivary Flow Rate in Clinical Types of Oral Lichen Planus. *Skinmed* **2018**, *16*, 19–22. [PubMed]
67. Lopez-Jornet, P.; Zavattaro, E.; Mozaffari, H.R.; Ramezani, M.; Sadeghi, M. Evaluation of the salivary level of cortisol in patients with oral lichen planus: A meta-analysis. *Medicina* **2019**, *55*, 213. [CrossRef] [PubMed]
68. Nadendla, L.K.; Meduri, V.; Paramkusam, G.; Pachava, K.R. Association of salivary cortisol and anxiety levels in lichen planus patients. *J. Clin. Diagn. Res.* **2014**, *8*, ZC01. [CrossRef] [PubMed]
69. Rödström, P.-O.; Jontell, M.; Hakeberg, M.; Berggren, U.; Lindstedt, G. Erosive oral lichen planus and salivary cortisol. *J. Oral Pathol. Med.* **2001**, *30*, 257–263. [CrossRef] [PubMed]
70. Koray, M.; Dülger, O.; Ak, G.; Horasanli, S.; Üçok, A.; Tanyeri, H.; Badur, S. The evaluation of anxiety and salivary cortisol levels in patients with oral lichen planus. *Oral Dis.* **2003**, *9*, 298–301. [CrossRef]
71. Stojanovich, L. Stress and autoimmunity. *Autoimmun. Rev.* **2010**, *9*, A271–A276. [CrossRef] [PubMed]
72. Wei, W.; Sun, Q.; Deng, Y.; Wang, Y.; Du, G.; Song, C.; Li, C.; Zhu, M.; Chen, G.; Tang, G. Mixed and inhomogeneous expression profile of Th1/Th2 related cytokines detected by cytometric bead array in the saliva of patients with oral lichen planus. *Oral Surg. Oral Med. Oral Pathol. Oral Radiol.* **2018**, *126*, 142–151. [CrossRef]
73. Hodge, D.R.; Peng, B.; Cherry, J.C.; Hurt, E.M.; Fox, S.D.; Kelley, J.A.; Munroe, D.J.; Farrar, W.L. Interleukin 6 Supports the Maintenance of p53 Tumor Suppressor Gene Promoter Methylation. *Cancer Res.* **2005**, *65*, 4673–4682. [CrossRef]
74. Mozaffari, H.R.; Sharifi, R.; Sadeghi, M. Interleukin-6 levels in the serum and saliva of patients with oral lichen planus compared with healthy controls: A meta-analysis study. *Cent. Eur. J. Immunol.* **2018**, *43*, 103–108. [CrossRef]
75. Baggiolini, M.; Clark-Lewis, I. Interleukin-8, a chemotactic and inflammatory cytokine. *FEBS Lett.* **1992**, *307*, 97–101. [CrossRef]
76. Mozaffari, H.R.; Sharifi, R.; Mirbahari, S.; Montazerian, S.; Sadeghi, M.; Rostami, S. A systematic review and meta-analysis study of salivary and serum interleukin-8 levels in oral lichen planus. *Postep. Dermatol. Alergol.* **2018**, *35*, 599–604. [CrossRef] [PubMed]
77. Rhodus, N.L.; Cheng, B.; Myers, S.; Miller, L.; Ho, V.; Ondrey, F. The feasibility of monitoring NF-κB associated cytokines: TNF-α, IL-1α, IL-6, and IL-8 in whole saliva for the malignant transformation of oral lichen planus. *Mol. Carcinog.* **2005**, *44*, 77–82. [CrossRef] [PubMed]
78. Rhodus, N.L.; Cheng, B.; Bowles, W.; Myers, S.; Miller, L.; Ondrey, F. Proinflammatory cytokine levels in saliva before and after treatment of (erosive) oral lichen planus with dexamethasone. *Oral Dis.* **2006**, *12*, 112–116. [CrossRef] [PubMed]
79. Warnakulasuriya, S. Global epidemiology of oral and oropharyngeal cancer. *Oral Oncol.* **2009**, *45*, 309–316. [CrossRef] [PubMed]
80. Mehrtash, H.; Duncan, K.; Parascandola, M.; David, A.; Gritz, E.R.; Gupta, P.C.; Mehrotra, R.; Amer Nordin, A.S.; Pearlman, P.C.; Warnakulasuriya, S.; et al. Defining a global research and policy agenda for betel quid and areca nut. *Lancet Oncol.* **2017**, *18*, e767–e775. [CrossRef]
81. Yete, S.; D'Souza, W.; Saranath, D. High-Risk Human Papillomavirus in Oral Cancer: Clinical Implications. *Oncology* **2018**, *94*, 133–141. [CrossRef]
82. Scheifele, C.; Reichart, P.A. Is there a natural limit of the transformation rate of oral leukoplakia? *Oral Oncol.* **2003**, *39*, 470–475. [CrossRef]
83. Offidani, A.; Simonetti, O.; Bernardini, M.L.; Alpagut, A.; Cellini, A.; Bossi, G. General Practitioners' Accuracy in Diagnosing Skin Cancers. *Dermatology* **2002**, *205*, 127–130. [CrossRef]
84. Mignogna, M.D.; Fedele, S.; Russo, L.L.; Ruoppo, E.; Muzio, L.L. Oral and pharyngeal cancer: Lack of prevention and early detection by health care providers. *Eur. J. Cancer Prev.* **2001**, *10*, 381–383. [CrossRef]
85. Mehdipour, M.; Shahidi, M.; Manifar, S.; Jafari, S.; Mashhadi Abbas, F.; Barati, M.; Mortazavi, H.; Shirkhoda, M.; Farzanegan, A.; Elmi Rankohi, Z. Diagnostic and prognostic relevance of salivary microRNA-21, -125a, -31 and -200a levels in patients with oral lichen planus—A short report. *Cell. Oncol.* **2018**, *41*, 329–334. [CrossRef]

86. Park, N.J.; Zhou, H.; Elashoff, D.; Henson, B.S.; Kastratovic, D.A.; Abemayor, E.; Wong, D.T. Salivary microRNA: Discovery, characterization, and clinical utility for oral cancer detection. *Clin. Cancer Res.* **2009**, *15*, 5473–5477. [CrossRef]
87. Sun, Y.-M.; Lin, K.-Y.; Chen, Y.-Q. Diverse functions of miR-125 family in different cell contexts. *J. Hematol. Oncol.* **2013**, *6*, 6. [CrossRef] [PubMed]
88. Ishikawa, S.; Sugimoto, M.; Edamatsu, K.; Sugano, A.; Kitabatake, K.; Iino, M. Discrimination of oral squamous cell carcinoma from oral lichen planus by salivary metabolomics. *Oral Dis.* **2020**, *26*, 35–42. [CrossRef] [PubMed]
89. Ma, B.; Simala-Grant, J.L.; Taylor, D.E. Fucosylation in prokaryotes and eukaryotes. *Glycobiology* **2006**, *16*, 158R–184R. [CrossRef] [PubMed]
90. Miyoshi, E.; Moriwaki, K.; Nakagawa, T. Biological Function of Fucosylation in Cancer Biology. *J. Biochem.* **2008**, *143*, 725–729. [CrossRef] [PubMed]
91. Sanjay, P.; Hallikeri, K.; Shivashankara, A. Evaluation of salivary sialic acid, total protein, and total sugar in oral cancer: A preliminary report. *Indian J. Dent. Res.* **2008**, *19*, 288–291. [PubMed]
92. Dhakar, N.; Astekar, M.; Jain, M.; Saawarn, S.; Saawarn, N. Total sialic acid, total protein and total sugar levels in serum and saliva of oral squamous cell carcinoma patients: A case control study. *Dent. Res. J.* **2013**, *10*, 343–347.
93. Dadhich, M.; Prabhu, V.; Pai, V.; D'Souza, J.; Harish, S.; Jose, M. Serum and salivary sialic acid as a biomarker in oral potentially malignant disorders and oral cancer. *Indian J. Cancer* **2014**, *51*, 214–218.
94. Panda, M.; Rai, A.K.; Rahman, T.; Das, A.; Das, R.; Sarma, A.; Kataki, A.C.; Chattopadhyay, I. Alterations of salivary microbial community associated with oropharyngeal and hypopharyngeal squamous cell carcinoma patients. *Arch. Microbiol.* **2019**. [CrossRef]
95. Healy, C.M.; Moran, G.P. The microbiome and oral cancer: More questions than answers. *Oral Oncol.* **2019**, *89*, 30–33. [CrossRef]
96. Marttila, E.; Uittamo, J.; Rusanen, P.; Lindqvist, C.; Salaspuro, M.; Rautemaa, R. Acetaldehyde production and microbial colonization in oral squamous cell carcinoma and oral lichenoid disease. *Oral Surg. Oral Med. Oral Pathol. Oral Radiol.* **2013**, *116*, 61–68. [CrossRef]
97. Marttila, E.; Uittamo, J.; Rusanen, P.; Lindqvist, C.; Salaspuro, M.; Rautemaa, R. Site-specific acetaldehyde production and microbial colonization in relation to oral squamous cell carcinoma and oral lichenoid disease. *Oral Surg. Oral Med. Oral Pathol. Oral Radiol.* **2015**, *119*, 697–699. [CrossRef] [PubMed]
98. Alnuaimi, A.D.; Ramdzan, A.N.; Wiesenfeld, D.; O'Brien-Simpson, N.M.; Kolev, S.D.; Reynolds, E.C.; McCullough, M.J. Candida virulence and ethanol-derived acetaldehyde production in oral cancer and non-cancer subjects. *Oral Dis.* **2016**, *22*, 805–814. [CrossRef] [PubMed]
99. Moritani, K.; Takeshita, T.; Shibata, Y.; Ninomiya, T.; Kiyohara, Y.; Yamashita, Y. Acetaldehyde production by major oral microbes. *Oral Dis.* **2015**, *21*, 748–754. [CrossRef] [PubMed]
100. Wu, J.; Peters, B.A.; Dominianni, C.; Zhang, Y.; Pei, Z.; Yang, L.; Ma, Y.; Purdue, M.P.; Jacobs, E.J.; Gapstur, S.M.; et al. Cigarette smoking and the oral microbiome in a large study of American adults. *ISME J.* **2016**, *10*, 2435–2446. [CrossRef] [PubMed]
101. Corbaux, C.; Joly, P. Bullous Diseases. In *Current Problems in Dermatology*; KARGER: Basel, Switzerland, 2017; Volume 53, pp. 64–69. ISBN 1421-5721.
102. Murrell, D.F.; Peña, S.; Joly, P.; Marinovic, B.; Hashimoto, T.; Diaz, L.A.; Sinha, A.A.; Payne, A.S.; Daneshpazhooh, M.; Eming, R.; et al. Diagnosis and Management of Pemphigus: Recommendations by an International Panel of Experts. *J. Am. Acad. Dermatol.* **2019**. [CrossRef] [PubMed]
103. Andreadis, D.; Lorenzini, G.; Drakoulakos, D.; Belazi, M.; Mihailidou, E.; Velkos, G.; Mourellou-Tsatsou, O.; Antoniades, D. Detection of pemphigus desmoglein 1 and desmoglein 3 autoantibodies and pemphigoid BP180 autoantibodies in saliva and comparison with serum values. *Eur. J. Oral Sci.* **2006**, *114*, 374–380. [CrossRef]
104. Ali, S.; Kelly, C.; Challacombe, S.J.; Donaldson, A.N.A.; Bhogal, B.S.; Setterfield, J.F. Serum and salivary IgG and IgA antibodies to desmoglein 3 in mucosal pemphigus vulgaris. *Br. J. Dermatol.* **2016**, *175*, 113–121. [CrossRef]
105. Hallaji, Z.; Mortazavi, H.; Lajevardi, V.; Tamizifar, B.; Amirzargar, A.; Daneshpazhooh, M.; Chams-Davatchi, C. Serum and salivary desmoglein 1 and 3 enzyme-linked immunosorbent assay in pemphigus vulgaris: Correlation with phenotype and severity. *J. Eur. Acad. Dermatology Venereol.* **2010**, *24*, 275–280. [CrossRef]

106. De, D.; Khullar, G.; Handa, S.; Joshi, N.; Saikia, B.; Minz, R.W. Correlation between salivary and serum anti-desmoglein 1 and 3 antibody titres using ELISA and between anti-desmoglein levels and disease severity in pemphigus vulgaris. *Clin. Exp. Dermatol.* **2017**, *42*, 648–650. [CrossRef]
107. Russo, I.; Saponeri, A.; Michelotto, A.; Alaibac, M. Salivary samples for the diagnosis of Pemphigus vulgaris using the BIOCHIP approach: A pilot study. *In Vivo* **2017**, *31*, 97–100. [CrossRef] [PubMed]
108. Brito-Zerón, P.; Baldini, C.; Bootsma, H.; Bowman, S.J.; Jonsson, R.; Mariette, X.; Sivils, K.; Theander, E.; Tzioufas, A.; Ramos-Casals, M. Sjögren syndrome. *Nat. Rev. Dis. Prim.* **2016**, *2*, 16047. [CrossRef] [PubMed]
109. Pasoto, S.G.; Adriano de Oliveira Martins, V.; Bonfa, E. Sjögren's syndrome and systemic lupus erythematosus: Links and risks. *Open Access Rheumatol. Res. Rev.* **2019**, *11*, 33–45.
110. Fernández-Martínez, G.; Zamora-Legoff, V.; Hernández Molina, G. Oral health-related quality of life in primary Sjögren's syndrome. *Reumatol. Clínica (Engl. Ed.)* **2019**. [CrossRef]
111. Ben-Chetrit, E.; Fischel, R.; Rubinow, A. Anti-SSA/Ro and anti-SSB/La antibodies in serum and saliva of patients with Sjogren's syndrome. *Clin Rheumatol.* **1993**, *12*, 471–474. [CrossRef] [PubMed]
112. Ching, K.H.; Burbelo, P.D.; Gonzalez-Begne, M.; Roberts, M.E.P.; Coca, A.; Sanz, I.; Iadarola, M.J. Salivary anti-Ro60 and anti-Ro52 antibody profiles to diagnose Sjogren's Syndrome. *J. Dent. Res.* **2011**, *90*, 445–449. [CrossRef]
113. Hu, S.; Vissink, A.; Arellano, M.; Roozendaal, C.; Zhou, H.; Kallenberg, C.G.M.; Wong, D.T. Identification of autoantibody biomarkers for primary Sjögren's syndrome using protein microarrays. *Proteomics* **2011**, *11*, 1499–1507. [CrossRef]
114. Ohyama, K.; Moriyama, M.; Hayashida, J.-N.; Tanaka, A.; Maehara, T.; Ieda, S.; Furukawa, S.; Ohta, M.; Imabayashi, Y.; Nakamura, S. Saliva as a potential tool for diagnosis of dry mouth including Sjögren's syndrome. *Oral Dis.* **2015**, *21*, 224–231. [CrossRef]
115. Kang, E.H.; Lee, Y.J.; Hyon, J.Y.; Yun, P.Y.; Song, Y.W. Salivary cytokine profiles in primary Sjögren's syndrome differ from those in non-Sjögren sicca in terms of TNF-α levels and Th-1/Th-2 ratios. *Clin. Exp. Rheumatol.* **2011**, *29*, 970–976.
116. Katsiougiannis, S.; Wong, D.T.W. The Proteomics of Saliva in Sjögren's Syndrome. *Rheum. Dis. Clin. N. Am.* **2016**, *42*, 449–456. [CrossRef]
117. Lee, J.; Lee, J.; Baek, S.; Koh, J.H.; Kim, J.-W.; Kim, S.-Y.; Chung, S.-H.; Choi, S.S.; Cho, M.-L.; Kwok, S.-K.; et al. Soluble siglec-5 is a novel salivary biomarker for primary Sjogren's syndrome. *J. Autoimmun.* **2019**, *100*, 114–119. [CrossRef]
118. Tandon, M.; Gallo, A.; Jang, S.-I.; Illei, G.G.; Alevizos, I. Deep sequencing of short RNAs reveals novel microRNAs in minor salivary glands of patients with Sjögren's syndrome. *Oral Dis.* **2012**, *18*, 127–131. [CrossRef] [PubMed]
119. Pauley, K.M.; Stewart, C.M.; Gauna, A.E.; Dupre, L.C.; Kuklani, R.; Chan, A.L.; Pauley, B.A.; Reeves, W.H.; Chan, E.K.L.; Cha, S. Altered miR-146a expression in Sjögren's syndrome and its functional role in innate immunity. *Eur. J. Immunol.* **2011**, *41*, 2029–2039. [CrossRef] [PubMed]
120. Alevizos, I.; Alexander, S.; Turner, R.J.; Illei, G.G. MicroRNA expression profiles as biomarkers of minor salivary gland inflammation and dysfunction in Sjögren's syndrome. *Arthritis Rheum.* **2011**, *63*, 535–544. [CrossRef] [PubMed]
121. Ibáñez-Cabellos, J.S.; Seco-Cervera, M.; Osca-Verdegal, R.; Pallardó, F.V.; García-Giménez, J.L. Epigenetic Regulation in the Pathogenesis of Sjögren Syndrome and Rheumatoid Arthritis. *Front. Genet.* **2019**, *10*, 1104. [CrossRef]
122. Konsta, O.D.; Thabet, Y.; Le Dantec, C.; Brooks, W.H.; Tzioufas, A.G.; Pers, J.O.; Renaudineau, Y. The contribution of epigenetics in Sjögren's Syndrome. *Front. Genet.* **2014**, *5*, 71. [CrossRef] [PubMed]
123. Thabet, Y.; Le Dantec, C.; Ghedira, I.; Devauchelle, V.; Cornec, D.; Pers, J.-O.; Renaudineau, Y. Epigenetic dysregulation in salivary glands from patients with primary Sjögren's syndrome may be ascribed to infiltrating B cells. *J. Autoimmun.* **2013**, *41*, 175–181. [CrossRef]
124. Baldini, C.; Giusti, L.; Ciregia, F.; Da Valle, Y.; Giacomelli, C.; Donadio, E.; Ferro, F.; Galimberti, S.; Donati, V.; Bazzichi, L.; et al. Correspondence between salivary proteomic pattern and clinical course in primary Sjögren syndrome and non-Hodgkin's lymphoma: A case report. *J. Transl. Med.* **2011**, *9*, 188. [CrossRef]
125. Cui, L.; Elzakra, N.; Xu, S.; Xiao, G.G.; Yang, Y.; Hu, S. Investigation of three potential autoantibodies in Sjogren's syndrome and associated MALT lymphoma. *Oncotarget* **2017**, *8*, 30039–30049.

126. Sharma, D.; Sandhya, P.; Vellarikkal, S.K.; Surin, A.K.; Jayarajan, R.; Verma, A.; Kumar, A.; Ravi, R.; Danda, D.; Sivasubbu, S.; et al. Saliva microbiome in primary Sjögren's syndrome reveals distinct set of disease-associated microbes. *Oral Dis.* **2019**. [CrossRef]
127. Siddiqui, H.; Chen, T.; Aliko, A.; Mydel, P.M.; Jonsson, R.; Olsen, I. Microbiological and bioinformatics analysis of primary Sjögren's syndrome patients with normal salivation. *J. Oral Microbiol.* **2016**, *8*, 31119. [CrossRef]
128. Li, B.; Selmi, C.; Tang, R.; Gershwin, M.E.; Ma, X. The microbiome and autoimmunity: A paradigm from the gut–liver axis. *Cell. Mol. Immunol.* **2018**, *15*, 595–609. [CrossRef] [PubMed]
129. Campanati, A.; Ganzetti, G.; Giuliodori, K.; Marra, M.; Bonfigli, A.; Testa, R.; Offidani, A. Serum levels of adipocytokines in psoriasis patients receiving tumor necrosis factor-α inhibitors: results of a retrospective analysis. *Int. J. Dermatol.* **2015**, *54*, 39–45. [CrossRef] [PubMed]
130. Campanati, A.; Ganzetti, G.; Giuliodori, K.; Postacchini, V.; Liberati, G.; Azzaretto, L.; Vichi, S.; Guanciarossa, F.; Offidani, A. Homocysteine plasma levels in psoriasis patients: our experience and review of the literature. *J. Eur. Acad. Dermatol. Venereol.* **2015**, *29*, 1781–1785.
131. Ganzetti, G.; Campanati, A.; Santarelli, A.; Pozzi, V.; Molinelli, E.; Minnetti, I.; Brisigotti, V.; Procaccini, M.; Emanuelli, M.; Offidani, A.; et al. Periodontal disease: an oral manifestation of psoriasis or an occasional finding? *Drug Dev. Res.* **2014**, *75*, S56–S59.
132. Ganzetti, G.; Campanati, A.; Santarelli, A.; Pozzi, V.; Molinelli, E.; Minnetti, I.; Brisigotti, V.; Procaccini, M.; Emanuelli, M.; Offidani, A. Involvement of the oral cavity in psoriasis: Results of a clinical study. *Br. J. Dermatol.* **2015**, *172*, 282–285. [CrossRef] [PubMed]
133. Ganzetti, G.; Campanati, A.; Santarelli, A.; Sartini, D.; Molinelli, E.; Brisigotti, V.; Di Ruscio, G.; Bobyr, I.; Emanuelli, M.; Offidani, A. Salivary interleukin-1β: Oral inflammatory biomarker in patients with psoriasis. *J. Int. Med. Res.* **2016**, *44*, 10–14. [CrossRef]

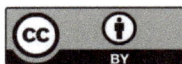

© 2020 by the authors. Licensee MDPI, Basel, Switzerland. This article is an open access article distributed under the terms and conditions of the Creative Commons Attribution (CC BY) license (http://creativecommons.org/licenses/by/4.0/).

MDPI
St. Alban-Anlage 66
4052 Basel
Switzerland
Tel. +41 61 683 77 34
Fax +41 61 302 89 18
www.mdpi.com

Journal of Clinical Medicine Editorial Office
E-mail: jcm@mdpi.com
www.mdpi.com/journal/jcm

www.ingramcontent.com/pod-product-compliance
Lightning Source LLC
LaVergne TN
LVHW070045120526
838202LV00101B/638